Social Work with Immigrants

People whose work brings them into contact with immigrants and their families are concerned about the serious personal and social problems they may face in establishing themselves in Britain. Originally published in 1972, Juliet Cheetham here explores the origin and nature of these difficulties and discusses the contributions and limitations of social work in meeting the needs of immigrants, their relatives and some of the organizations involved with them at the time.

Drawing on her own field experience, the author deals with fundamental issues in race relations, together with the problems of poor urban areas in which most immigrants have settled. She also considers the backgrounds of some of the main immigrant groups, their family structure, and the pressures and anxieties they experience in moving into a new environment. She examines as well the special skills and understanding that social workers in this field need to develop.

This is a perceptive study which raised fundamental questions about the values, objectives and methods of social work at the time. Even today it will also provide social workers with a stimulus to re-think the basis of some of their activities.

This book is a re-issue originally published in 1972. The language used, and assumptions made, are a reflection of its era and no offence is meant by the Publishers to any reader by this re-publication.

Social Work with Immigrants

Juliet Cheetham

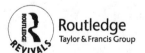

Routledge
Taylor & Francis Group

First published in 1972
by Routledge & Kegan Paul Ltd

This edition first published in 2022 by Routledge
2 Park Square, Milton Park, Abingdon, Oxon OX14 4RN

and by Routledge
605 Third Avenue, New York, NY 10158

Routledge is an imprint of the Taylor & Francis Group, an informa business

Publisher's Note
The publisher has gone to great lengths to ensure the quality of this
reprint but points out that some imperfections in the original copies may
be apparent.

Disclaimer
The publisher has made every effort to trace copyright holders and
welcomes correspondence from those they have been unable to contact.

A Library of Congress record exists under ISBN: 0710073658

ISBN: 978-1-032-11287-9 (hbk)
ISBN: 978-1-003-21926-2 (ebk)
ISBN: 978-1-032-11293-0 (pbk)

Book DOI 10.4324/9781003219262

Social Work with Immigrants

Juliet Cheetham

Lecturer in Applied Social Studies,
University of Oxford

LONDON AND BOSTON
ROUTLEDGE & KEGAN PAUL

TO PAUL

First published 1972
by Routledge & Kegan Paul Ltd,
Broadway House, 68-74 Carter Lane,
London EC4V 5EL and
9 Park Street,
Boston, Mass. 02108, U.S.A.
Printed in Great Britain by
Northumberland Press Limited,
Gateshead
© Juliet Cheetham 1972
ISBN 0 7100 7365 8 (c)
          7366 6 (p)
Library of Congress Catalog Card Number: 72-81443

General editor's introduction

se . . we . . . . . . written the web of the problems . . . . know what to do things f and . . . . chapter, but the author respect with for we need clearly useful . . . a guide that follows a static . . . . . .

The Library of Social Work is designed to meet the needs of students following courses of training for social work. In recent years the number and kinds of training have increased in an unprecedented way. The Library will consist of short texts designed to introduce the student to the main features of each topic of enquiry, to the significant theoretical contributions so far made to its understanding, and to some of the outstanding problems. Each volume will suggest ways in which the student might continue his work by further reading.

As Juliet Cheetham says, 'Very little has been written about social work with immigrants and practically nothing that is relevant to the UK'. Her book admirably fills this gap, not because it could be said 'to give social workers all the answers' (whatever they might be) to the problems social workers are increasingly acknowledging, but because it helps us to see some of the main questions that should be posed and pressed against an informed and broadly conceived background. The author begins, rightly in my view, with problems of definition and with the story of recent policy in connection with immigration, pointing out its double-edged nature—imposing controls and slowly recognizing the place of specialized provision. This is followed by two chapters of detailed discussion of the social circumstances of immigration and the strains of migration; the place and point of social work is shown by means of general discussion and case illustration—if it is true that social work readers of other kinds of book ignore the statistical tables, I hope that other kinds of reader will not skip these realistic and helpful illustrations. Chapter 5 is concerned with the social and cultural background of certain groups of immigrant, and this often seems to social workers the hub of the problem: once we are informed about social and cultural sources we shall know what to do. There is useful information in this chapter, but the author begins with the warning, equally useful, against assuming that culture is static and failing to take account of adaptations made, willingly or unwillingly, to migration. Finally, problems of method and policy are examined in a way that marks the attainment of the main aim of this book, 'to help social workers to think about these questions which must be studied in greater depth in the next few years'.

This book has a place in the Library of Social Work for three main reasons. Firstly, it attempts to relate social work directly to a range of problems, without assuming that social work can offer all the solutions or that rather narrow boundaries have to be maintained around the subject in order to ensure it can be managed. The limitations of social work (community work as well as casework) and its possibilities for real usefulness are recognized even though migration 'must be seen in the context of gross differences in the wealth of nations' and even though in our present situation 'immigrant' is often a by no means neutral equivalent for 'black', with all the complexity entailed in that term. Secondly, the book stresses the importance of good information without denying problems in the application of such knowledge. Problems of the interpretation of the facts (hence the author's early delineation of the frameworks of the stranger, social class, and minority group) and of the changing nature of the facts are crucial in this and in all other areas of social work. Thirdly, the subject of this book makes a contribution to the continuing debate in social work about generic and specific elements. The author does not ignore elements in the problems connected with migration that are common to other situations, but we are helped to see the special problems and to appreciate that an increasingly refined perception of them is in no sense 'discriminatory'.

NOEL TIMMS

Contents

CONTENTS

Acknowledgments

This book grew out of my experiences of working with immigrants in London and I would like to express my gratitude to all the people who talked to me about their lives with such patience and perception; I hope that what I have written reflects my affection and regard for them.

I am also grateful to my colleagues in social work, too numerous to mention by name, who have shared with me their own experience of work with immigrants.

The general editor, A. H. Halsey, Jenny Hammond, Michael Hill, and Olive Stevenson read the manuscript and I am greatly indebted to them for giving me so much of their time and for their valuable criticism and encouragement.

My thanks are also due to Mrs Sylvia Boyce and Mrs Jackie Evans for their patience and skill in deciphering and typing the final draft of the manuscript.

Most of all, I am grateful to my husband who bore the brunt of my anxiety and preoccupation while this book was being written.

1

Some definitions and problems

Migration is central to human experience. The search for a promised land which would be a refuge and a home for the poor and oppressed and the opportunities of gaining wealth and power by colonial expansion have always drawn people to seek their fortunes outside their native countries. This has been achieved by the settlement of under-developed territories, by the sale of labour in countries whose expansion depended on manpower they did not possess themselves, and by conquest and exploitation. All migrants experience some hardship, and even when they are welcomed and needed, their presence is usually accompanied by tensions which can become the concern of politicians and administrators. In recent years, social workers in many countries have also been concerned with immigrants and this has involved them not only with their welfare but also, implicitly or explicitly, with the protection of those interests of the receiving society which may be threatened by newcomers. American and Israeli experience provide numerous examples of these dual and sometimes conflicting preoccupations. British social workers are now also facing these challenges and it is their contact with immigrants with which this book is chiefly concerned.

For centuries Britain's wealth of natural resources, her expanding industries, and to some extent her liberal, political, and religious ideals have attracted those whose security has been threatened in their native countries.

Attitudes towards these immigrants and the treatment they have received have been influenced by Britain's perception of the reasons for their migration, her view of their social and cultural background and, most important, her understanding of the kind of contribution they were likely to make to their new country.

At various times public concern has been expressed about the number of immigrants coming to the UK and the conditions in which they chose or were forced to live. The Aliens Act of 1905, designed to restrict the entry of poor Russian and Polish Jews, and the Commonwealth Immigrants Acts of 1962 and 1968 are indications that the initial sympathy extended to victims of political or religious persecution or the notion of the rights in Commonwealth citizenship are tempered very much by Britain's perception of what appear to be her own immediate interests. In the latter case the loss of imperial power and the reassessment of the role of the Commonwealth contributed to a perception of these interests largely in domestic terms. Although the economic contribution of immigrants to Britain has been recognized, there has also been considerable alarm about the consequences of the presence, mainly in urban areas, of large numbers of coloured people coming mainly from the 'New' Commonwealth, that is all Commonwealth countries with the exception of Australia, Canada, and New Zealand. This concern has been present in demands both for the strict control of immigration, particularly that of coloured people, and for policies to protect and promote their interests. The following chapters will show how muddled these measures have been, and how this confusion has been reflected in the contact social workers have had with immigrants.

The shape of these policies and the priority they assume must be understood in the context of assumptions about the rights and needs of immigrants and their place in British society. Although some of these attitudes are present in any country which has experienced immigration on a large scale, others arise directly from the philosophy and beliefs which have traditionally permeated British social policies and are further influenced by her experience of imperial power.

Some conceptual frameworks

1 *The immigrant as a stranger* The simplest and most unsophisticated view of the immigrant is that of the stranger lost in an alien but not necessarily unwelcoming world, who will, in the course of time, find his feet in his new situation. This perception, often including the assumption that the immigrant will return soon to his native country, asks that some allowance should be made for unfamiliarity with the customs of a new country and for the reserve and possible mild antipathy of the native population in the face of this. The onus is on the new-comer to find a place for himself in society, even if only on its fringes. If he does not return home, it is assumed that he, or anyway his children, will gradually assimilate to the new country. These assumptions, which rely very much on *laissez-faire* principles, underly the assertions, characteristic until the last decade of British policy towards immigrants, that no special efforts should be made to meet their needs. They ignore the many social and economic pressures which militate against the acceptance of the 'stranger' as an equal, especially if his cultural background is very unfamiliar, and also the wishes of some immigrants to preserve their national identity at the same time as they press for equality of treatment. This perception of immigrants will be blind to the various attempts which are nearly always made, consciously or unconsciously, to exclude them from sharing the rights and privileges enjoyed by the majority of the native population.

2 *Immigrants and the working class* Another perception

3

of the immigrant is of a person whose recent arrival and willingness to take any employment, no matter what its conditions, place him, at least temporarily, in the lowest strata of society, so sharing their frustrations and deprivations. This view is well founded in fact. Traditionally, immigrants, many of whom are unskilled, have sought and accepted a role as a replacement labour force living in the least favoured areas vacated by those who are successfully pursuing better jobs and living conditions. However, because of their industry and their willingness to endure considerable hardship in their efforts to establish themselves socially and economically, many immigrants to Britain, especially those from Europe and Ireland, have achieved a substantial degree of social mobility. This achievement has lessened fears about the formation of a permanent alien working-class minority and accounts for the view that any problems that immigrants might experience, because of their similarity with those of the deprived working class, demand the same treatment.

Most studies of coloured or white immigrants and the areas in which they first settle have revealed not only hardships and deprivations shared with the poor working class but also the way in which the presence of immigrants draws attention to these problems. Some have also shown how the demands of urban life and competition for the scarce resources of the most deprived areas lead to an inevitable conflict of interests and the exclusion, sometimes deliberate, of some of the weakest members of society from a share of the few good things of life and their exploitation by the more powerful. Amongst those falling behind in this struggle will be families with young children, unsupported mothers, and other people whose personal circumstances and poverty leave them with little bargaining power. Those who are unfamiliar with urban life and have problems of adjustment in a new society will also be vulnerable.

There are, however, other factors which ensure that

some immigrants have little chance of improving their circumstances. The most potent of these is discrimination which excludes them, more or less permanently, from all but the most menial and poorly paid jobs, the worst housing, and consequently the most inadequate amenities and social services. In a competitive and deprived environment this discrimination has its roots in beliefs that some people, perhaps because of the way they conduct their lives, or because as newcomers they should be at the end of the queue for employment, housing, and welfare, are not fit for or should not share in the rights and privileges hoped for but infrequently received by the rest of the community. Groups of people who are readily identifiable, especially if they are unfamiliar, can also serve as useful scapegoats, and because they are seen as the cause of the ills of society, they are still further excluded from its benefits.

Most immigrants are to an extent identifiable and so can expect to experience discrimination, the ill effects of which are often tempered by their resilience and perseverance. In time, their increasing familiarity with the life of their new country and their adaptation to it makes many immigrants, and certainly their children, indistinguishable from the rest of the community. However, those immigrants who are coloured and therefore the most easily identifiable may continue to experience discrimination and exploitation whatever their personal circumstances and however long their stay in the new country. As a result, they and their children can be firmly trapped in a deprived environment from which it is hard to escape both because they are barred from superior employment and housing and because their surroundings provide few opportunities for advancement.

Evidence of the extensive discrimination experienced by coloured people is irrefutable. In an illuminating book, Rex (1970) has argued that this prejudice arises partly because of certain stereotyped views concerning their incapacity to achieve social advancement. Consequently, they are seen as outside and beneath the stratified system of society. Sometimes these views have their roots in beliefs about the innate inferiority of certain races but, in a European context, they are most often the inheritance of colonialism and slavery whose systems of dominance and control over black people were largely incompatible with ideas about their actual or potential equaliy with the white races.

Mason (1970) has described how the differences in various colonial systems have influenced contemporary perception and treatment of colonized people. For example, the paternalism of British colonialism, which saw its subject people as eventually maturing sufficiently to run their own affairs and benefiting from adopting some of the laws and traditions of their masters, can still be detected in attitudes towards immigrants in the UK. However, no colonial system has escaped, and most have encouraged, the age-old association of blackness with inferiority. In a country like Britain, with such a recent imperial history, few people can be unaware of this association.

It has also been argued that some people are especially likely to be racially prejudiced if their personalities predispose them towards aggression, particularly against minority or unfamiliar groups, a reliance on strict control of individual freedom, and severe sanctions for deviant behaviour. This group will include some who feel they have failed in many important respects in their emotional and social lives and who will be tempted to see the presence of newcomers as contributing to their failure. Since these personality traits are present to some extent in all people and cannot be associated exclusively with one distinguishable group, this view of prejudice cannot, on its own, account for the many different ways in which it will be expressed, including the active discrimination of one group or individual against another. This can most usefully be understood in the context of the social and economic environment.

The presence of coloured immigrants in the most deprived areas, drawing attention to the problems of the inner city and highlighting the struggle for scarce resources and the inevitable conflict, together with certain views of coloured people as alien and inferior, should, therefore, temper the relatively optimistic view that they are members in all important respects of the poor working class and likely only temporarily to face discrimination which hampers their social mobility. There is already some evidence that coloured people, whether they are old established immigrants or born in the UK are finding it difficult or even impossible to achieve the acceptance and social and geographical distribution which would normally be expected given the length of their residence in Britain.

There are some serious problems inherent in this perception of coloured people as potentially the weakest, most deprived, and most frustrated members of the poor working class. If it became clear that the extent of discrimination against them was such that they were particularly at risk of being trapped indefinitely in a vicious circle of poor opportunity and poor attainment, special measures which positively discriminated in their favour might be necessary, either to prevent their entry into this vicious circle or to help them to escape from it. Because such treatment would be resented and envied by poor whites, the tension between them and coloured people could be increased. Consequently, there are as yet few demands for the privileged treatment of coloured people and any special efforts that are made on their behalf are not usually openly acknowledged or encouraged. The emphasis is on reducing actual or potential conflict between white and coloured people both by focusing on their common problems and uniting them in solving these and by restricting the over-all numbers of coloured people in Britain. Some efforts, so far largely unsuccessful, have also been made to prevent their concentration in some of the poorest areas. It is not yet clear how successful these policies will be and in spite of the obvious dangers of such measures, if the emergence of a grossly deprived and frustrated coloured minority seemed likely, its special and priority needs would have to be recognized and met.

3 *Immigrants and minority groups* The third perception of immigrants is as members of minority groups, aware of their separate identity, with their own internal hierarchy, and anxious to preserve their own cultural traditions. Such groups may have a degree of self-sufficiency which involves them only in minimal contact with the native community. They ask for little more than the right to work and to be left in peace to pursue their own way of life. Some Jewish, Pakistani, and Indian immigrants can be seen as following this pattern of self-sufficiency and voluntary isolation. But after the earliest stages of migration, competition and conflict with the wider environment tend to increase. Few immigrants who are aware of their own national or cultural identity will consciously seek assimilation with the native community. More usually, with the rising expectations that come after a few years settlement in the new country, they ask for the civil rights, and social and economic benefits accorded to the native population as well as respect for their own traditions and measures to safeguard them.

Although there is a risk that focusing on minority groups will encourage the view that some people are potentially always an alien irritant in society, in many respects, this view of immigrants is an attractive one. It underlies one of the most popular definitions of integration not as a process of assimilation involving the loss by immigrants of their own national characteristics and culture but as 'equal opportunity accompanied by cultural diversity, in an atmosphere of mutual tolerance' (Jenkins, 1966). However, it cannot be assumed that 'mutual tolerance' and cultural diversity will accompany each other if one group feels deeply that its own interests will thereby be threatened. It is probably more realistic to expect conflict between groups seeking some degree of acceptance and equality of treatment and those who are anxious for various reasons to exclude them from this, and to explore ways of reducing or managing that conflict. This is achieved sometimes by reducing the economic and political power of the weaker groups and sometimes by providing a legal framework for the expression of conflict and sometimes by providing for social and economic equality. It can also mean fostering each group's awareness of its own identity and interests so that it can negotiate with the other from the basis of some security. Such security may arise from feelings of confidence associated with membership of organizations offering full acceptance to their members, a familiar environment and objectives which are immediately sympathetic to them.

In recent years policies affecting immigrants in Britain have been accompanied by some attempts to allow for the needs and wishes of different immigrant groups although there is a prevailing assumption that their children will not want or be able to maintain these distinctions to any great extent. Immigrants are expected to abide by the laws of the country and to accept some of its customs, although the extent to which they should be required to do this is frequently a matter of dispute. When the security and protection of minority groups are seen as providing their members with a springboard into the wider community, they are now usually welcomed and accepted by those who bear responsibility at local and national level for policies affecting immigrants. However, if minority groups are seen to be encouraging membership and cohesion largely for the purpose of pursuing their own exclusive interests, they frequently give rise to considerable anxiety.

The popularity of each of the three perceptions we have been considering depends partly on prevailing social and economic philosophies. Each one has something to contribute to an understanding of immigrants and the treatment they receive. It is not always easy to see which is most influential in determining British attitudes and policy, including those of social workers, although currently the view of coloured immigrants as particularly vulnerable members of the working class seems to predominate. This is reflected both in the expectations that they, like all who share the deprivations of life in the poorest areas, will benefit from the extra efforts made to alleviate them, and in the assumption that they place an added strain on the social services and so their numbers should be restricted. At the same time, attempts have been made to protect the interests of coloured people in legislation designed to decrease discrimination. In recent years it has also proved increasingly helpful to understand immigrants in the context of their different national and cultural backgrounds and to be aware of the implications of the maintenance of these special identities in Britain.

The role of social work

The future of immigrants and their children depends largely on far reaching policies designed to alleviate the problems of the most deprived members of society whatever their social background. These policies involve the redistribution of resources, the planning and rebuilding of some urban areas, and the safeguarding of the rights of minority groups. The contribution of social work to these policies and to the welfare of immigrants is a small but important one.

Firstly, social work should be concerned to help the small minority of immigrants with serious personal or social problems. It is unlikely that the number of these will be large, partly because many immigrants belong to the twenty to thirty-five age group, which makes few demands on the social services, and partly because of the resourcefulness and perseverance which characterize most immigrant groups. None the less, the strains of migration are great and the following chapters will describe some of the problems of living in the poorest areas, of loss and adjustment to a new society of which newly arrived immigrants are acutely aware, and the conflict they experience in their families and with the native population. Social work has something to offer in the alleviation of these difficulties. One of its strengths lies in a flexibility of approach arising from the importance attached to understanding the particular circumstances surrounding individual problems and the development of personal relationships with those who need help. This sometimes makes it possible for social workers to adapt or interpret general policies to meet individual needs in a realistic and helpful way.

Another and more general contribution of social workers should be the provision of information about the problems facing minority groups and the adequacy or inadequacy of the social services which exist to solve them. Social workers are often amongst the first of those in authority to know of these difficulties, and in the course of their work some have the opportunity for longer and closer relationships with immigrants and their families than most members of the native population. Ideally, therefore, they should in some cases be able to act as a bridge between immigrants and natives, interpreting the one to the other when difficulties and misunderstandings arise and, where appropriate, working for a modification of behaviour and attitudes.

For various reasons, social workers have not always been equal to these demands. Their recent preoccupation with individual pathology rather than the economic problems and poor environment of many of their clients means that some do not identify, understand, or offer appropriate help to many of those in need. The present trend in social work towards giving more material and practical aid and increasing involvement in community work could alter this state of affairs.

More specifically, some social workers have found it hard to understand and even to sympathize with the problems of their immigrant clients. For example, the attitudes of some immigrants towards their children seems excessively strict and even punitive to English social workers. Not surprisingly, many immigrants are confused by the complexity of the social services and often neither understand nor sympathize with their aims. This has sometimes led to impatience on the part of social workers rather than sustained attempts at explanation or efforts to evolve ways of working which will be more helpful to immigrants. It should also be recognized that, however much they may wish to deny it, social workers may share the prejudices of the rest of the population and some will feel hostile towards immigrants. This antagonism will obviously affect their work with them although it will probably not be openly expressed.

Many social workers now recognize these shortcomings and are asking for information about immigrants' social and cultural background and their lives in Britain. There is also a demand for reassessment of social work methods in relation to the particular difficulties of immigrants as well as the ones shared with those living in deprived areas.

The scope and limitations of this book

This short book is intended to give some help to those concerned with these questions, but it has several limitations. Space prevents discussion of all but the most recent immigrants to the UK, particularly those from India. Pakistan, and the West Indies, and of the work being done by British social workers, whereas a comprehensive study would include consideration of immigration and social work services in many countries, especially the USA and Israel. There are, however, many similarities in the problems and needs of all immigrants whatever their nationality or ethnic origin and wherever they decide to settle. Although the main focus of this book is social work with coloured immigrants, much of what is written applies also to white immigrants.

Very little has been written about social work with immigrants and practically nothing that is relevant to the UK. However, a great deal of information has recently been collected about the social conditions of coloured immigrants and their families in Britain, and one aim of this book is to discuss the implications of this information for social work. Another purpose is to look at the knowledge and social work skills which are most useful in work with immigrants and to discuss possible adaptation. The focus here will be mainly on issues common to all methods of social work and not on a detailed examination of the contributions of these different methods, partly because of limitations of space, but also because there is a lack of information in England about the appropriate use of methods other than social casework. So far, little is known about how immigrants of different backgrounds understand and use the social services, what sort of treatment they receive from social workers, and whether social services or methods of work should be evolved to meet their needs. This book aims to help social workers to think about these questions which must be studied in greater depth in the next few years.

Some general problems

1 *The definition of immigrant* For many people the word 'immigrant' is synonomous with coloured. They ignore the fact that large numbers of coloured people living in Britain were born here, and the frequent use of the term 'second-generation immigrant' can denote a lack of acceptance of coloured people as citizens of the UK. The Department of Education and Science defines an

'immigrant' child as one who was born outside this country or who was born to parents who were themselves not born in the UK and who have lived here less than ten years. In enlarging the literal meaning of 'immigrant', the Department is recognizing that special consideration should also be given to the children of immigrants; and by excluding children from the Republic of Ireland in the compilation of statistics relating to immigrant children, the Department is also implying that particular account should be taken of 'coloured' immigrant children and those who might be expected to have language difficulties.

2 *Some objections to the special consideration of immigrants* The advisability of focusing particularly on the problems of immigrants may be questioned. Some people think that to discuss a problem may define and crystallize it beyond hope of solution. On the other hand, there are those who, relying on *laissez-faire* principles, believe that it is wisest not to interfere with problems which in the course of time will sort themselves out. There are also those who think that looking at problems presented by immigrants will, by recognizing differences, imply prejudice or discrimination. In addition, there is the fear that an examination of these problems could lead to an acknowledgment that existing services may be inadequate to cope with them. These beliefs lay behind the reluctance of departments, until very recently, to compile statistics relating to immigrants' use of their services. These attitudes, however well meaning, have not been in the interests of either immigrants or the rest of the population. The absence of information has meant that some of the real problems of immigrants have either been ignored or exaggerated and ignorance about numbers of immigrants has led to wild speculation and fear that the social services will be flooded with requests for help. Social workers, as well as many other people who are concerned with immigrants, are now recognizing that here ignorance is not bliss.

3 *Positive discrimination* The discussion of the special needs of immigrants is also feared by those who think that it is unwise or undesirable to give special attention to a minority group, particularly a coloured minority group, which cannot be given to the rest of the population. This anxiety reflects the conflict facing politicians and social administrators over the provision of universal or selective services. Some minority groups have only recently succeeded in becoming priority groups, and the Plowden Report of 1967, *Children and their Primary Schools*, marked the advent of policies involving positive discrimination in the allocation of resources in favour of areas where there is serious deprivation. This concept of positive discrimination contradicts the belief that the definition of particular areas or problems implies negative attitudes and policies.

None the less, the treatment of special needs raises difficult questions, familiar to social workers, about the liberty of the individual and the right to equality of treatment. For example, in their work with immigrants, social workers may have to decide whether the criteria for taking their children into care should be the same as those for the native population. Should special recognition be given to the needs and wishes of many immigrant mothers to work full time and the consequent risks involved in private fostering? If coloured children are taken into care, should special arrangements be made for them to maintain contact with coloured people? Questions of this kind have only recently been asked by social workers. Although there are no clear answers to them, this book will discuss some issues they raise.

Some social workers are reluctant to make distinctions between the needs of coloured immigrant clients and those of native clients. They believe that their familiarity with European and Irish immigrants and general experience of working with an increasingly mobile population and of helping people to understand and use appropriately a bewildering number of social services, will stand them in good stead whatever the ethnic background of their clients. While it is helpful to identify common problems and approaches, it should not be assumed that the existing knowledge and expertise of social work are equal to all its tasks. This complacency has harmed both social workers and their clients. At a time when they are being given more resources and more responsibilities, social workers must be aware that new approaches may be needed in work with groups of people whose problems and backgrounds are unfamiliar. Immigrants and their families are only one of these groups.

4 *The problem of the isolation of special groups* Social workers are rightly cautious of attempts to isolate groups of individuals according to their apparent state, rather than their real needs. Divisions of responsibility in social services which were based on differences between those in need—i.e. the delinquent, the handicapped, the mentally ill, the poor, and the homeless—have proved in many cases to be unhelpful. It would be most unfortunate if the consideration of the special needs of coloured immigrants implied that these needs are in themselves quite different to those of the rest of the population. Any attempt to study and provide for the needs of different groups must take into account the benefits and dangers implicit in specialization; but nevertheless, some special awareness of particular problems can be a necessary and helpful step towards providing flexible services of a high standard.

2

Background, policies, and numbers

Comparisons are often made between the three major immigrant groups which have come to Britain in the last hundred years, the Russian and Polish Jews, the Irish, and the New Commonwealth immigrants. Although the absence of comparable statistical information makes exact comparisons impossible, there are some similarities in the reception, treatment, and settlement of the various groups, at least in the early years of their migration. There are also indications of special factors associated with immigration from the New Commonwealth. Although this most recent immigration covers a span of only twenty years—which makes it hard to discern with accuracy the patterns of settlement amongst coloured immigrants and their families—it has been relatively well documented and there are signs that the geographical and social mobility of these New Commonwealth immigrants will be more limited than that of European and Irish immigrants.

European and Irish immigrants

Immigrants from Ireland and from Russia and Poland in the early part of the century have never made up more than about 2 per cent of the whole population. The proportion of Irish immigrants is slightly larger in certain urban areas, particularly London and the Midlands. Both the Irish and the Jews, at least initially, sought security and protection in the company of their compatriots; and in the early years of the century, their living and employment conditions were frequently appalling. Both groups, especially the less familiar European Jews, have attracted hostility. However, partly because their contribution to the economy, has been valued—particularly in the case of the Irish—their presence has been tolerated and their civil rights protected, although the government has made no special attempts to assist or promote their settlement or integration in Britain. Fears have sometimes been expressed that these immigrants will swamp the social services with their demands but although the settlement of some Irish families has presented problems, both they and the Jews have proved themselves to be resourceful people often turning in need to voluntary organizations, sometimes founded by themselves. Neither the Irish nor the Jews have ever represented a major political lobby except possibly in some rather limited urban areas.

Although these Irish and Jewish immigrants came mainly as poor unskilled labourers, they or their descendants have achieved a high degree of social and geographical mobility, which supports the view that immigrants share only temporarily the deprivations of the poor working class. The Russian and Polish immigrants were helped to establish themselves by the existing Jewish community in England, and in the course of two or three generations their descendants seem to have achieved a position in society similar, if not somewhat superior, to the rest of the population. While some have maintained Jewish cultural and religious practices, their original national identity is of no importance and they see themselves, and are seen, as British citizens.

The position of the Irish is somewhat different, partly because among the steady flow of new immigrants from Ireland, there are many who will take unskilled jobs and settle in some of the poorest areas on their arrival in Britain. Many Irish also remain here only temporarily and their continued contact with Ireland contributes to an awareness of some degree of special identity amongst Irish immigrants. However, the census shows that the Irish are widely distributed socially and geographically. Although there is no way of ascertaining the social class of the children of Irish immigrants, this relatively wide distribution amongst their parents would suggest a fair degree of social mobility. Their position in British society is interesting in that they stand mid-way between the native population and the recent immigrants from the New Commonwealth.

Immigration from the Commonwealth

Until the Second World War immigrants from Commonwealth countries were largely descended from those who had left the UK to settle in the Dominions and Colonies or those who were returning home after a period of duty abroad. They were therefore nearly all white. The few coloured Commonwealth citizens living in Britain were traders, students, or diplomats. The war-time experiences of many members of the armed forces seem to have left them with a wish to emigrate and the post-war years witnessed a heavy flow of migration within the Commonwealth. Many people left the UK to settle in Australia, Canada, and New Zealand; and in addition, West Indians, Indians, and Pakistanis, many of whom had travelled extensively during the War, decided to emigrate to Britain, at that time one of the few major industrial nations not strictly controlling immigration, or to other Commonwealth countries.

The post-war rebuilding programme in Britain and the expansion of the economy meant that there was a heavy demand for all kinds of labour—a demand that was not fully met by Irish and European immigrant workers. From the 1950s, large numbers of coloured Commonwealth citizens began to arrive in the UK. This demand for labour coincided in some cases with comparatively poor economic conditions in the Commonwealth countries. However, Peach (1968) has shown that it was the fluctuations of the British economy and not the economic conditions of the Caribbean which largely determined the rise and fall of West Indian immigration during the 1950s. There is little reason to suppose that immigration from other Commonwealth countries such as India and Pakistan was influenced by very different factors. To a large extent the immigrants from the Commonwealth, like other immigrants before them, have acted as a replacement population. They have gone to areas where there has been a continuing demand for labour but a declining population since employment in these areas has often not proved attractive or lucrative enough for native labour. London and the South East, which for many years have attracted both immigrant and native labour, are exceptions to this rule.

Some new anxieties

The concentration of large numbers of coloured immigrants in areas where amenities were inadequate, drew attention to the fact that although economic conditions favoured immigration, social conditions, in particular the shortage of housing, did not. The belief that the Welfare State was all-embracing and all-providing was severely shaken by the realization during the late 1950s and early 1960s that services were severely strained and also that many people were either not being reached by existing services or were not benefiting from them. While some people assumed, quite mistakenly, that control of immigration from the Commonwealth would do much to ease the strain on the social services, there were others who were anxious, with greater justification, about the concentration of poor families, both white and coloured, in some of the most deprived urban areas. The somewhat naïve belief that the British people, with a tradition of Commonwealth and colonial interests, would understand and tolerate coloured people, was also not well founded. Competition for scarce resources, particularly housing, resulted in fear and tension amongst those living in the poorest urban areas. Though there was little overt violence between the white and coloured inhabitants of these districts, it was clear that coloured immigrants were not only becoming scapegoats, blamed as the source of all the problems in the area, but were also facing severe discrimination in their search for employment, housing, and other services. Some observers began to forecast an outbreak of conflict similar to that in many American cities if the number of coloured people in Britain increased significantly and if no measures were taken to protect their interests and improve the conditions of all those living in the most deprived areas.

This situation, combined with fears of an economic recession, a growing nationalism, and some disillusionment with the Commonwealth, influenced the British government to remodel its immigration policy.

The statistics of Commonwealth immigration

Between 1955 and 1962 numbers of immigrants from the New Commonwealth coming to the UK varied between 21,000 and 57,000 annually. Fears of possible restrictions on immigration account for the increase in numbers in the months immediately preceding the passing of the Commonwealth Immigrants Act in 1962 after which numbers decreased steadily to under 30,000 in 1970. The great majority of these immigrants are dependants, many of whom are coming to join relatives who came to Britain before the imposition of controls; as more families are reunited, the total numbers of Commonwealth immigrants will decrease further, assuming immigration regulations do not change.

Since the 1961 Census, special efforts have been made to record the number of immigrants from the New Commonwealth permanently resident in the UK, the areas in which they live, and such other information as their housing conditions, family size, and socio-economic status. In 1966 a special record was kept of the children of immigrants from the New Commonwealth and the 1971 Census has asked for information about the birth-place of the parents of all those living in Britain. However, it is at present difficult to estimate the size of the coloured as opposed to the immigrant population and variations in fertility rates also make it hard to predict accurately its growth, although there have been some methodical attempts to do this.

Using material from the 1966 10 per cent Sample Census, the Institute of Race Relations' 'Survey of Race Relations in Britain' (Rose *et al.*, 1969) has estimated that in 1966 the main coloured groups were:

Caribbeans	454,000
Indians	223,600
Pakistanis	119,700
	797,300

These figures exclude white people born in India and Pakistan, but include the children of coloured immigrants who were born in Britain. Rose *et al.* (1969) also calculated that there were rather less than a million Commonwealth immigrants from the New Commonwealth and coloured British born in England and Wales, slightly less than 2 per cent of the total population. In the absence of more current census data, the suggested total for 1969 is 1,185,000 which takes into account estimates of births and net arrivals (Deakin, 1970). The coloured population is predominantly youthful and in 1966 it was estimated that 34 per cent of all coloured immigrants (including their children born in the UK) were under fifteen, and 55 per cent were aged between fifteen and forty-five. Those who are in employment are mostly grossly over-represented in the lowest socio-economic groups and the limited social and educational opportunities of many of the children of immigrants, plus the discrimination they face in the search for employment, make it unlikely that their occupational status will be substantially different during the next twenty years.

Immigrants from the Commonwealth and their families are not evenly distributed throughout Britain. They have gone to areas of traditional immigrant settlement, that is, London, some seaports, and towns where there is a heavy demand for unskilled labour. Nevertheless, in 1966, in no town did immigrants from the New Commonwealth represent more than 5 per cent of the total population. In the great majority of towns less than 2 per cent of the population were coloured immigrants. The pattern for London is similar although in a few boroughs immigrants from the New Commonwealth make up between 5 and 7 per cent of the total population.

These numbers may be compared with those for alien and Irish immigrants. The 1966 Census found that there were over 800,000 foreign-born people living in England and Wales and nearly 700,000 who had been born in Eire; and it has been estimated that more Irish than Commonwealth immigrants come to Britain each year. There are, therefore, only small differences in the size of all the major immigrant groups in the UK. However, this has not prevented the immigration of coloured people from becoming the major focus of concern, largely because these immigrants have been seen as a peculiarly foreign group, readily identifiable because of their colour, whose settlement in Britain is likely to constitute a long and difficult process.

New immigration policies

From about 1960 the control of immigration was fiercely

debated. In the absence of hard information about coloured immigrants, speculation was rife both about their numbers and about the conditions in which they lived. The crucial issue was seen to be the need for control of immigration, particularly the immigration of coloured people. The control of Irish immigration was never seriously contemplated. There was no suggestion at this time that special services should be provided either for immigrants or for the improvement of the poor conditions prevailing in the areas where most coloured immigrants lived.

The Commonwealth Immigrants Act eventually became law in 1962. Its provisions are complicated, but its most important intention was to restrict immigration from the Commonwealth to those possessing employment vouchers and to the wives and children under sixteen of those either possessing vouchers or already in Britain. There were three types of voucher: A vouchers for Commonwealth citizens who had a specific job waiting for them in the UK, B vouchers for those possessing a recognized skill or qualification which was in short supply, and C vouchers for all other applicants, issued mainly on a 'first come, first served' basis. The number of vouchers issued annually was to be fixed by the government, taking into account factors such as the employment situation in Britain and pressures on the social services.

Debate did not end with the Act. In 1965 the issue of C vouchers was discontinued and the number of A and B vouchers reduced to 8,500 annually. The White Paper which announced these proposed changes also outlined government proposals to assist integration into what was described as a 'multi-racial society'. These proposals included a general attack on the housing shortage rather than special aid for immigrants, some limited help for local authorities where a large number of immigrants lived, support for the principle already proposed by the Ministry of Education that the proportion of immigrant children in any school should not exceed one-third, and

24

the setting up of the National Committee for Commonwealth Immigrants. The main work of the NCCI was to expand and improve the services of the local voluntary committees whose aim was to establish good relations between the immigrants and native population. The White Paper also referred to the discrimination experienced by many Commonwealth immigrants seeking employment and suggested measures which should be taken to counter it. However, the Race Relations Act, which was also passed in 1965 and prohibited discrimination on racial grounds in places of public resort and in the disposal of tenancies, did not extend to employment.

In 1971 a new Immigration Act was passed which, amongst other measures, limits right of entry to Britain to 'patrials', i.e. to those whose parents were citizens of the UK, usually because they were born in the British Isles. This effectively excludes immigrants from the New Commonwealth who will only be able to enter the UK to take up specific employment. Once in Britain their period of stay will be subject to restrictions in that work permits will usually be issued initially for a period of one year, although these may be renewed for a period of three years. Furthermore, Commonwealth immigrants who do not have patrial status will have no right to bring their dependants to the UK although the Home Secretary has indicated that permission to accompany or join those holding work permits may be granted to wives and to those children under sixteen whose parents are both living in Britain. The Act also makes provision to pay the travelling expenses of non-patrials who wish to return to their native countries. These regulations, most of which are likely to come into effect in 1972, will not apply to immigrants who, after five years' residence in Britain, have decided to take out, by registration, citizenship of the United Kingdom and Colonies. Nevertheless, it seems likely that the intention and spirit of the Act will harm race relations in so far as it contributes to the feelings of insecurity and rejection amongst coloured people in Britain.

'Double-edged' policies

The year 1965 marked the first time that the British government adopted a dual policy towards immigration, negative in the sense of imposing further controls and positive in its recognition, albeit somewhat limited, of the special needs of immigrants. This double-edged policy characterizes legislation and measures affecting race relations in many countries. In Britain it was continued in 1968, when, on the one hand, further restrictions were imposed on the entry of immigrants from the Commonwealth and, on the other, the scope of the Race Relations Act was extended to cover discrimination in employment and in the provision of goods and services. In addition, the Community Relations Commission, a new statutory body with an increased budget and greater authority, took over the functions of the NCCI. The main function of the Community Relations Commission is the establishment of harmonious community relations, and it is empowered to advise and make recommendations to the Home Secretary. In 1968 the government also announced its urban aid programme under which it authorized special expenditure on housing, education, health, and welfare in areas of special social need. A substantial degree of immigrant settlement was one of the factors to be considered in the definition and selection of these areas.

Many people regret this apparently almost inevitable combination of positive and negative policies, believing it to satisfy the interests of neither the native nor the immigrant populations. In particular, they are critical of what they consider to be the very paltry measures taken by the government to improve the conditions which prevail in the more deprived urban areas as it is the alleviation of these problems which is crucial to the establishment of good community relations.

26

Not surprisingly, this mixture of policies is viewed with some suspicion and ambivalence by immigrants. The clear unwillingness of the government and the public to tolerate a substantial increase in the coloured population, combined at times with suggestions of repatriation for some immigrants, are not necessarily countered by efforts to protect the rights of minority groups, even when it is obvious that their life chances are in most cases much poorer than those of the rest of the population.

The involvement of social workers

Social workers need to take account of this pattern of positive and negative measures present in both local and national policies and its implications for the people with whom they work. For example, some local education authorities have decided to disregard school catchment areas and to disperse coloured immigrant children throughout the schools in a certain area. The purpose of this policy is to avoid too great a concentration of coloured children in any one school and to make it easier to cater for the particular needs of immigrant children, such as language teaching. While some of these authorities do arrange special small classes for newly arrived immigrant children or those whose English is poor, it has to be admitted that this policy of dispersal has been adopted partly to relieve the fears of many white parents that their children would suffer if they were educated in schools where the majority of children were coloured. They fear, as do teachers and administrators, that 'black' schools will be bad schools.

Social workers are familiar with this kind of anxiety and hostility which can reflect both irrational prejudice and the tensions of competition for scarce resources. They know it will not disappear in the course of reasonable discussion and that other measures may have to be taken to avoid a potentially difficult situation. On the other hand, they will also be in touch with coloured people who may view this policy of dispersal with ambivalence or hostility. While wanting good educational facilities for their children, they are deeply suspicious of the selection of children for dispersal on the grounds of colour rather than any special needs they may have. They resent the assumption that too great a proportion of coloured children can lead to a decline in standards and be a focus of local hostility and conflict. They may also regret that their children are educated far from home. West Indian immigrants have a further source of resentment in that a higher proportion of their children, compared to white children, are deemed to be educationally subnormal and placed in special schools. They feel, with considerable justice, that even though the intentions of educational authorities may be good, they often fail to recognize that intelligence tests are culturally biased and so give an inaccurate estimate of a West Indian child's ability. They also think that, in many cases, few attempts are made to cater for the special needs of West Indian children in the context of the normal school and see the disadvantages of special schooling as out-weighing its advantages.

Social workers need to be aware of the tensions of the areas in which they work and they cannot ignore the policies which may contribute to them. They should realize too that since most of them are employed by local authorities, they will be identified with their policies and this will obviously affect the attitudes of those with whom they work. Some social workers, particularly those involved in community work, may have a duty to help people to make their opinions about problems and policies known to local authorities and to press for solutions. Social workers may also think that it is right for them to make known their own collective knowledge and opinions about certain social problems. Whatever may be the special focus of their work, they must realize that their activities and opinions and the problems and attitudes of those with whom they work are shaped not only by prevailing social and economic conditions but also by local and national policies. They cannot be politically innocent or indifferent.

3

The social circumstances of immigration

In so far as this immigration [from the New Commonwealth] has had its problems, particularly in the field of housing, education, health and welfare, these have been mainly in areas where difficulties in these fields have already been fairly marked ... they can be regarded as an additional symptom of an existing and more general problem—that of labour shortage, housing deficiency and the general social stress arising from continued concentration of employment and population in and around an already big, crowded and partly outworn urban complex' (Department of Economic Affairs, 1965, p. 53).

In the last few years a number of research studies have documented the social conditions experienced by immigrants and some of the poor native working class. These can only be briefly described and those who would like further information should turn to the suggestions for further reading listed in the final section of this book. These studies show the need for social workers to distinguish between those problems with which they can usefully concern themselves, and those which require large-scale political and economic intervention. There is at present an alarming tendency for the solution of complex social problems to be associated with the increased activities of social workers. If they collude with this naïve assumption, they may unintentionally mislead those with whom they work by giving them the impression that social work can do more to alleviate their difficulties than is actually the case. More important, by appearing to take responsibility for solving problems not within their competence, social workers can draw attention away from the real causes and the radical measures which may be needed to solve them. In their work with immigrants it is especially important for social workers to be aware of the implications of their activities.

Some characteristics of areas inhabited by immigrants

The previous chapter has described how immigrants have acted as a replacement population taking over the jobs, and sometimes the accommodation, which do not attract those who are in a position to choose where they live and work. This frequently entails residence in the decaying inner rings of large cities, some areas of which may be scheduled for redevelopment. The accommodation these areas offer usually consists of flats and rooms in Victorian houses or small terraced houses, whose few amenities make them relatively cheap to purchase.

These areas are sometimes described as ghettoes, as if they were entirely given over to coloured immigrants. This assumption of social or ethnic concentration seems to be made partly because the relative unfamiliarity of coloured people draws attention to them, and partly because immigrants, being young people, move outside their homes, in the course of their daily business, far more frequently than do the white residents who are often older and retired. It is therefore quite easy to assume from a casual glance at the people in the streets that these are coloured ghettoes. This is not an accurate description in terms of the numbers involved. Peach (1968) suggests that in 1961 there were possibly a few enumeration districts in which coloured people were in the majority and that since then they may have come to form a majority in a few more districts. Though the degree of dispersal is unclear, there are no areas of any substantial size inhabited only by coloured people. Nevertheless, their increased concentration in deprived areas is likely if they continue to find the road to the more affluent suburbs blocked by discrimination in employment and in housing and house purchase.

Some observers now see these areas not as immigrant but problem ghettoes. Clustered together in the rooms and flats of large houses, formerly the homes of prosperous merchants, are many people whose need for accommodation is desperate and who, for a variety of reasons, are not able to obtain accommodation in other areas. They include immigrants of all races and couples with young children, too poor to obtain a mortgage or unfurnished accommodation, or too newly arrived in a town to be eligible for a council house. Also finding shelter in these houses are people with particular problems, including unsupported mothers, discharged prisoners, ex-psychiatric patients and those whose deviant behaviour forces them to live on the fringes of society. These people are not welcome in more affluent districts even if they are able to find accommodation there.

These areas have been described as 'zones of transition' since many people living in them intend to move out as their circumstances improve. But amongst the shifting population are many who are unable to obtain better accommodation in more prosperous districts and who can move only within these deprived neighbourhoods. A number of factors including housing shortages and inadequate welfare policies contribute to the concentration, and indeed the segregation, of many people whose need for adequate accommodation and good social services is very great in the areas least equipped to provide them.

Few professional people are attracted to work where amenities are so poor; local authorities are reluctant to spend money on improving or even maintaining houses and roads in areas scheduled for clearance and redevelopment. Those medical and welfare services which must be available by statute are not so well equipped or serviced as in other more affluent or newly established districts. Most teachers do not want to work in overcrowded schools, perhaps with a constant flow of children who stay for only brief periods and whose economic, emotional, and intellectual deprivation gives rise to difficult and chronic problems. Lawyers, whose services are often greatly needed, do not usually wish to practice in these districts. Nor do the areas attract large-scale business such as supermarkets and other chain stores which can both add a prosperous air to a neighbourhood and provide goods and services at more competitive prices than smaller firms.

Anyone who gives these areas more than a cursory glance will be aware of their drabness, the general air of decay, the depression which grips a district which was at one time favoured and prosperous and of which its residents are now ashamed. And yet, by the present standards of local government they cannot be immediately cleared and redeveloped either because conditions are not seen as bad enough to justify this or because it would be impossible to rehouse the large numbers of people made homeless by these schemes. Furthermore, large-scale investment is usually not thought worthwhile. They therefore seem to be forgotten, to be the responsibility of no one, neither living under the immediate threat or hope of redevelopment nor worth the attention which could improve their amenities. They are districts in limbo, in the words of Rex and Moore (1967, p. 29), 'twilight zones which have not yet reached the night of slumdom'.

Jostling for position in these neighbourhoods are many older residents, some of whom may have been there all their lives. They may bitterly resent the declining standards and be full of nostalgia for a past which they remember as prosperous and gracious. In some cases they attribute this decline to the immigrants, white or coloured with whom, as the most recent newcomers to the area,

33

they associate its obvious problems of overcrowding, poverty, and poor facilities. Resenting the fact that they have been left behind in the exodus to greater prosperity, these older residents feel deserted, left to fight a losing battle against the decline of their neighbourhood, often torn between withdrawing completely or expressing open hostility to those whom they hold responsible for their troubles.

In these districts there is an absence of communal institutions and traditions which could give security to the older residents and act as a model for the newcomers. They are provided neither by the long-established residents, most of whom are elderly couples whose children have left home, nor by the many disparate immigrant groups whose energy is primarily directed towards survival and, sometimes, an escape to more congenial surroundings. The loyalty of many newcomers towards these areas will therefore be minimal. Although their age and needs make them potentially the most likely people to press for improved amenities by political and other means, at least in the early days of their settlement, they have little energy or inclination to do this. The anxiety, bitterness, and frustration engendered by life in such deprived neighbourhoods makes tension more probable than co-operation amongst its residents. They are unlikely to be able to identify their common interests and may interpret their problems in racial terms.

Immigrants and housing

Although immigrants have been seen as the cause of the housing shortage, most people in authority now accept that they are amongst its most vulnerable victims. The Milner Holland Report (1965) described the pressures on newcomers to live in central urban areas and their inevitable inheritance of overcrowding and poor facilities; Burney's (1967) graphic account of the housing problems shared by young families and newcomers to any large town, illustrates the way in which immigrants expose the failure of Britain's social, economic, and political institutions to meet the needs of her weakest citizens and minority groups.

Rose (1969) and Deakin (1970) describe in some detail the special housing problems of immigrants. They show that in Greater London and the West Midlands, where 60 per cent of all coloured immigrants live, they can expect substantially worse overcrowding than the native population in the least favoured accommodation. A far greater proportion have to contend with the problems of shared dwellings with communal facilities, and, between 1961 and 1966, when these problems decreased amongst the native population, they increased amongst coloured immigrants.

Only a few coloured immigrants enjoy the security of tenure which goes with unfurnished accommodation, and a tiny minority are housed by local authorities. Not all immigrants, particularly Indians and Pakistanis, want to rent local authority accommodation; but some, including a number of West Indians, would like this opportunity, although they are frequently not aware of the procedures surrounding its allocation. Furthermore, many boroughs have imposed lengthy conditions of residence on those born outside the UK before they are eligible even for local authority waiting lists. This practice has now been declared unlawful by the Race Relations Board and the Cullingworth Report (1969), in drawing attention to the special needs of immigrants, re-emphasized the principle of allocation of council housing according to need and recommended that there should be no residential qualification for admission to a housing waiting list. Even if these principles were accepted and put into practice immediately, and there seems little likelihood of this, large numbers of immigrants would still be at the end of the queue for local authority housing even though they may have lived in Britain for several years.

Amongst those immigrants who have managed to obtain local authority accommodation there is disturbing evidence that many have been allocated inferior houses, often patched dwellings bought up as part of slum clearance plans. There is a notable absence of immigrants on the newer and more prestigious housing estates. Although some immigrants may want the cheaper accommodation, Burney (1967) and other writers have shown how it can also be allocated to them because they are not aware of, and so do not ask for, the alternatives, and because Housing Visitors, believing the living standards of immigrants to be inferior, recommend that they should be allocated the poor quality housing.

The great majority of immigrants are therefore owner-occupiers or live in rented furnished accommodation. The purchase of a house is one of the chief ambitions of immigrant families, not only because it symbolizes their success and ability to establish themselves in a new country, but also because it is one of the most efficient ways of providing housing which is relatively secure and which can be adapted to suit their needs. However, the houses they can afford to buy are often old and somewhat dilapidated with only short leases remaining. The short-term loans and high rates of interest, which make their purchase possible, involve heavy repayments and sometimes these can only be met if owners let a number of rooms. Many immigrants also feel an obligation to provide accommodation for their relatives and friends. While some of these houses are overcrowded and the accommodation poor, with all the attendant possibility of conflict between landlord and tenant, these immigrant landlords provide an essential service to those for whom no other form of housing is available because of their colour, style of life, or insecure income. This service is frequently disregarded in criticism of the standard of accommodation offered. Rex and Moore (1967) have described how a city which has failed to solve its own housing problems, turns on those on whom it relies to make alternative provision and punishes them for their failure to do the job well in extremely difficult circumstances.

Probably some of the most fortunate immigrants are those who have been able to buy small cheap houses able to accommodate only one family and perhaps one or two lodgers, thus escaping the trials of multi-occupation. Although these houses often lack some basic amenities, immigrants take pride in caring for them and many are rescued from further deterioration by local authority improvement grants. Having security of tenure, their inhabitants are less mobile and, in areas with this type of accommodation, a mutually co-operative and friendly spirit can grow.

Finally, in their struggle to provide themselves with accommodation, coloured immigrants meet a problem not shared by the native population, that of discrimination against them on the grounds of colour. Of the studies that have revealed this, the most conclusive is the P.E.P. Report (1967) which has been summarized by Daniel (1968). This not only discovered substantial discrimination against coloured people in letting and house purchase, including the provision of mortgages and loans, but also found that the majority of immigrants do not expose themselves to this discrimination by looking for accommodation on the open market. This kind of discrimination has now been outlawed by the Race Relations Act 1968, but there are many loop-holes and it is not yet known how successfully the Act will achieve its objectives.

Immigrants and education

Using the definition of the Department of Education and Science, about 3 per cent of all school children are immigrants, with the largest numbers falling in the five to nine age group. Because the present age structure of the immigrant population means that they will have young children, this proportion will increase during the next decade. Furthermore, their concentration in certain urban areas, already described, means that a few schools will have large numbers of coloured children while the majority will have none. The controversy which surrounds their education, including the policy of dispersal described in chapter 1, is interesting as it reflects the attitudes of the government and public towards immigrants as a whole and highlights some of the differing ideals of the immigrant and native populations.

The failures and shortcomings of the British educational system have been well documented and much discussed in recent years. In particular, the Newsom Report (1963) and the Plowden Report (1967) drew attention to the inequalities and poor educational facilities available to many children in secondary modern schools and to those who go to primary schools where the buildings, the teaching available, and the social and emotional background of many children all combine to frustrate their development, grossly hampering their chances of using fully the existing facilities and of being selected for the best schools. Since immigrants live in many of the areas with the poorest amenities, disproportionate numbers of their children will go to the kind of schools about whose facilities the Plowden and Newsom Reports expressed the gravest reservations. The immigrant children who have come to these schools in fairly large numbers since the early 1960s have not caused the deterioration in standards and amenities which have been felt acutely in the last few years by teachers, parents, and children alike; but since some of them have special needs, they do place an extra burden on the teachers, especially when no attempt is made to meet their needs early in their school careers. As a result, the potential of many children is never realized.

This is a situation shared by many native children, and there is much more in the social and educational experience of native and immigrant children which is similar. The economic and cultural poverty of many of their homes, the strains on their parents which leave them little energy to involve themselves with their children's experiences in and out of school, and the general deprivation of the areas in which they live, make up a pattern which is familiar to many teachers and social workers. However, many immigrant children have some extra problems as well as some special advantages.

Some of the most severe problems are experienced by children who have spent some years in other countries before coming to Britain. The Plowden Report describes their situation well:

> They have often been abruptly uprooted, sometimes from a rural village community and introduced, maybe after a bewildering air flight, into crowded sub-standard housing in an industrial borough. This happens to European immigrants from Cyprus, Italy or Eire, as well as to the Commonwealth immigrants from the West Indies, parts of Africa, India or Pakistan. When the immigrant is Hindu or Muslim, and has special religious or dietary customs, difficulties for both child and teacher increase greatly. The worst problem of all is that of language. Teachers cannot communicate with parents; parents are unable to ask questions to which they may need to know the answers. It is sometimes impossible to find out even a child's age or medical history. Opportunities for misunderstandings multiply (p. 69).

When children uprooted in this way arrive in school, it is often difficult to distinguish a child with low intelligence and ability from one suffering from 'culture shock' and who needs to withdraw into himself as part of the process of adjustment. This is a time when a child may give quite a false impression of himself and it is easy to make wrong assessments of him.

In particular, the child who has already received part of his education abroad has special difficulties. It is likely that his previous educational experience will be dissimilar from what he finds in Britain. He may mistake the informal atmosphere of many schools for a total lack of discipline and be unaware of the values which are obvious or implicit to native children. He may react with wild and inappropriate behaviour, earning for himself sanctions which he does not understand or sees as unfair. Even if he has done well in his previous school, the different work, language problems, and a general feeling of confusion may mean he is unable to achieve similar success in his new school. Both he and his parents will be disappointed.

Most immigrant parents value education highly and are very anxious that their children should do well at school. Indeed, one of their reasons for immigration may have been to provide their children with good educational opportunities. They realize that only success is likely to make them acceptable to British society and that good educational attainment may help their children to escape the depressing environment which surrounds many immigrant families and breeds the vicious circle of low opportunities and low attainment to the third and fourth generations. These ambitions for their children mean that immigrant parents make great efforts to ensure that their children attend school regularly and have the proper equipment. They are also willing for them to stay on at school after the official school-leaving age in the hope that they will pass exams or obtain other qualifications.

Nevertheless, many immigrant parents are unimpressed and bewildered by aspects of the English educational system. They think the discipline is far too lax or non-existent, and see schools, particularly coeducational schools, as providing opportunities for their children to learn bad ways and become as ill-disciplined and disrespectful to their parents as English children. They doubt the educational value of many of the subjects in the curriculum and, in the words of one parent, they would prefer 'reading, writing, number and no nonsense'. In a study of Jamaica, Kerr (1957) has described educational experiences familiar to many West Indians who, in their native islands, have seen a place in school as a prized privilege, where discipline was harsh and much learning conducted by rote. Such experiences would make it difficult for them to understand English educational methods. These attitudes, combined with the social deprivation of many immigrant families, mean that their educational ideals cannot always bear fruit. The school can be a source of disruption and strain as well as achievement.

Unfortunately, it is not easy for many immigrant parents to communicate with teachers and make their views known. They may feel shy and overwhelmed by discussions in a school or else attract the disapproval and even the hostility of teachers if they express their views in a way which teachers see as inappropriate or unreasonable. Furthermore, teachers may feel far more sympathetic to immigrant children than to their parents whom they sometimes see as harsh disciplinarians making quite unrealistic demands on their children.

Immigrant children are likely to be aware of a clash of culture and custom both within school and outside. They will be torn between a wish to identify with their friends and share their privileges and way of life, and their loyalty to their parents who may wish them to retain, as far as possible, the culture of their native countries. The lack of communal institutions and traditions in the areas of transition in which so many immigrants live, and the disruption of the culture of the immigrant groups mean that their families are confused about the norms or standards of behaviour with which to identify. The schools in these areas may provide a rather hazy pattern of British culture but this is likely to have strong middle-class overtones and therefore seem alien to the majority of the pupils.

Immigrant families often have to live amongst families with many personal problems; however, they do not necessarily share these problems. When the background of immigrant children is more secure than that of native children, they may have a better chance of educational success. This is increased if they are ambitious and willing to work hard. So far there is little evidence from which to judge or predict the relative achievement of white and coloured school children although some studies suggest that the coloured children born in the UK do at least as well as white native children living in similar circumstances. Much will depend on their teachers' perception of their potential. Paradoxically, if they are seen as successes, this may cause conflict between white and coloured people. If it is no longer possible for coloured immigrants and their families to be cast as scapegoats and inferior beings, their success could add to the insecurity, envy, and hostility of the poor white working-class families who are their neighbours. Already teachers are aware that while there is little overt hostility or discrimination between white and coloured school children in primary and junior schools, this does appear, sometimes in quite acute forms, when children become adolescent. This may be because at this age children are more readily aware of the opinions of their parents and are influenced by their anxieties and prejudices; but, undoubtedly, some of this tension arises from the competition, real or supposed, amongst young people, about to leave school, who are looking for jobs.

It is in this context that the aspirations of immigrant parents and their children are frequently judged to be unreal and too high by teachers, social workers, and careers officers. Although some families may have unrealistic ambitions for their children as part of the apparently hopeless and desperate effort to improve substantially their position in society, some teachers and other officials are inclined to see nearly all the school leavers in certain areas as potential failures in terms of high status employment, and so are unlikely, often quite unfairly, to take seriously the aspirations of immigrant families. Beetham (1967) has described how some coloured children differ from many secondary modern school children whose modest ambitions are easily fulfilled and who therefore integrate fairly easily into the world of employment. Furthermore, the discrimination which seriously limits the number of jobs available to coloured school leavers, makes it tempting to see them as being fit only for those jobs open to them. In his autobiography, Malcolm X (1970) gives a horrifying account of his favourite teacher's failure to recognize his potential and his attempt to push him towards those low status jobs he thought befitted Negro boys.

Many schools are very concerned about the education and welfare of their coloured pupils but often find it difficult to establish contact with their parents. The teacher-social workers who are being appointed in some schools could have a valuable contribution to make here. Those social workers in touch with immigrant children who have particular problems and who can be a cause for serious concern in schools, need to work closely with teachers. They may sometimes be able to establish a closer relationship with immigrant parents than is possible for teachers and so may be more aware of the confusion, resentment, and disappointment which seem to be shared by many immigrants. Equally, they may be able to help parents to understand, and perhaps come to terms with, some aspects of the English educational system; sometimes they can help parents to accept that their children may not find the kind of employment or place in further education they had so much desired and for which they had worked so hard. A social worker may be able to act as a bridge between parents and teachers, and parents and children, provided she has taken time to understand their points of view. The following case provides an example of some of the strains experienced by immigrant parents and their children, and of the work which teachers and social workers were able to do together in their attempts to give them some partial relief.

Family and school in conflict: a case study

The Children's Department were consulted by the head-master of a mixed comprehensive school because he was most concerned about Nasreen Khan, a fourteen-year-old Pakistani girl. Although she was described as very with-drawn and shy, she had a good relationship with her class teacher and had confided in her that her father was ex-tremely strict with her, refusing to let her go out un-accompanied and never after she returned from school. She was apparently expected to do a number of domestic tasks including a great deal of the cooking for the immediate family as well as relatives. She was actively discouraged from doing homework, and said that her father was ex-tremely critical of the school and would have taken her away had he not been told that in doing so he would be breaking the law. Over a period of some months Nasreen became more listless and unhappy and eventually refused even to talk to her favourite teacher, although at one time she blurted out that her father was now involved in nego-tiations over her betrothal to a boy in Pakistan and that she might soon be returning to marry him.

The Children's Department learnt also that Nasreen's sixteen-year-old brother, Farrukh, although a highly intelli-gent boy, was not progressing as well as he should, and that in school his behaviour alternated rapidly between periods of intense concentration and periods of listless, apathetic withdrawal.

His parents were thought to be very ambitious for him but not very understanding about the time he had to spend on school work. Nor apparently were they very happy with his fairly independent thinking and wish for a more westernized life. Farrukh was also expected to act as a chaperon for Nasreen and interpreter for his many rela-tives, duties which he found tedious. The youngest child, Hassan, aged thirteen, was of average ability but, in spite of his parents' reservations about Farrukh's progress, under great pressure to do as well academically as his brother. His father had complained to the school about him, and indeed about the competence of the school, when his school reports were not as good as Farrukh's.

The staff of this school had already had some contact with these children's parents and other Moslem families over arrangements for their children to be withdrawn from Christian religious activities and for recognition of dietary laws. It had been agreed that Moslem girls should wear trousers with their school uniform and a separate room had been made available for their use when they were not in formal classes. Having made these special arrangements, most of the staff felt that the Moslem parents would have to make some adaptation by allowing their children a measure of independence and appreciating the difficulties of their life in two very different environments, at home and at school. They were especially concerned about Nasreen, particularly since she had hinted that she might have to return to Pakistan to a life which would now be very strange to her. The headmaster had visited her parents and there had been a rather acrimonious exchange during which each party had accused the other of neglecting the children in their charge, the headmaster saying that Nasreen's parents were not concerned for her welfare and development as an adolescent girl and her father accusing the school of compromising her virtue by allowing her to associate unsupervised with boys. He also said several times very angrily: 'You are stealing my boy and my girl—I will send them home. My family will not fall into bad ways'; to which the headmaster retorted that he would refer the whole matter to a higher authority. Nasreen's father had apparently seemed frightened by this, saying that he had never had any trouble with the police and that everyone was against his family because they were coloured.

Not surprisingly, the first contact of the woman Child Care Officer who visited the family, was very strained.

45

Although she made a point of visiting when both parents were present, she was put off by Mrs Khan referring all questions addressed to her, interpreted by a relative, to her husband. Mr Khan made some quite wild accusations against the school, adding that he thought his daughter was already 'spoilt'; no one would want to marry her and he would have to send her back to Pakistan where people would not know that she had associated with boys. He again repeated several times that 'people were stealing his children'. Nasreen and Farrukh were present during this discussion but took no part, and looked extremely uncomfortable especially when their father shouted at them that they had brought shame on their family. In addition, Hassan was accused of being lazy and ungrateful for all the sacrifices his parents had made for him to get a good education. The Child Care Officer tried to explain to Mr and Mrs Khan that she understood their anxieties, but was not very successful. She did, however, get the impression that Mr Khan was not only angry but hurt and frightened. He told her several times about the difficulties he had in establishing his family in Britain and concluded by asking what the police would do. He seemed rather astonished when told that the police had nothing to do with this matter and that the Child Care Officer had come to find out about their worries and why they felt so angry with the school. She wisely decided at this stage not to put forward the concerns of the teachers and asked if she could call again, saying she would like to hear about the family's life in Pakistan.

The atmosphere at subsequent visits was quite different and resembled that of a rather formal social occasion during which the Child Care Officer was plied with tea and cakes served by Nasreen, with Farrukh sitting in the background, clearly bored by the proceedings but under pressure from his parents to be there. The Child Care Officer at first doubted the value of these contacts and felt that the extreme politeness and reserve which characterized them obscured the real feelings of the family. The teachers continued to be concerned about Nasreen and Farrukh. However, the atmosphere gradually thawed. The Child Care Officer still wondered what was being achieved, but was pleased that the parents were now talking more freely about their life in the UK. They spoke movingly of their financial struggles to save enough money for their fares to Britain, to buy their terraced house, and to support their relatives in Pakistan. They thought it unlikely they would ever see their older children again and agreed that this made it all the more important to them that Nasreen, Farrukh, and Hassan should remain united with the family. Mr Khan spoke with indignation of the humiliation experienced by many coloured people in the UK and about the way he was treated at work, expected to do the hardest jobs and not welcomed in the union. He emerged as a dignified if somewhat rigid man whose support outside his family was in religious associations. Mr and Mrs Khan also discussed their views about some aspects of the English way of life of which they disapproved. The Child Care Officer did not always agree with them and although it seemed unlikely that she or they would change their opinions to any significant degree, there was a genuine exchange of ideas, an understanding and respect for each other's viewpoint. Mr and Mrs Khan said that the Child Care Officer was the first English person with whom they had been able to talk in this way.

Slowly a picture of the family's hopes, struggles, and fears emerged; and in the now peaceful and friendly atmosphere, Mr and Mrs Khan showed quite clearly that they were aware that their children's lives would be different from theirs, but were confused about how much freedom to allow them and very anxious lest there should be any fundamental break with Farrukh if, in going to technical college and qualifying as an engineer, he should be drawn away from his relatives. There was no further mention of Nasreen's return to Pakistan.

47

The Child Care Officer had made no attempt so far to talk to Nasreen and Farrukh alone as she guessed that their father's accusations that people tried to steal his children stemmed from fear that some people sympathized entirely with them without taking his feelings or opinions into account. However, she did have several discussions with the teachers explaining Mr and Mrs Khan's position and advising them, if possible, not to identify too closely with the children since, in the long run, this was likely to be unhelpful for them and their parents.

When the Child Care Officer eventually suggested to Mr and Mrs Khan that Nasreen might go to a club started at the school especially for Pakistani girls, they agreed readily and discussed the various possible activities with her and the headmaster who was by now seen in a much more friendly light. It was also agreed that Mrs Khan should attend an English class being held at the school for Pakistani women and the Child Care Officer arranged for her to travel there either with herself or a voluntary worker. Language difficulties prevented much discussion on these journeys and Mrs Khan remained a rather shadowy figure. However, it was clear that both the volunteer and the Child Care Officer were seen as trusted family friends and invited frequently to the Khan home. Mr Khan made himself responsible for telling other Pakistanis in the neighbourhood about these classes and under his sponsorship a number of other families made use of them.

Over a period of some months the teachers saw that Nasreen was far happier and more relaxed. Having been allowed some freedom, and realizing that her teachers and parents were not now in open conflict, she appeared to accept her somewhat confined life. Farrukh, however, was clearly in great doubt about his future and wondering how far some course of higher education would alienate him from his family. Nevertheless, he was now able to discuss this at some depth with his teacher and it seemed likely that he would go to technical college. Although this would

probably add to his ambivalence about his family's outlook and way of life, he seemed to be able to accept and
face this better now that it had been aired and discussed
to some extent with his parents. His class teacher made
quite a good relationship with them and it seemed probable
that their pride and delight in Farrukh's success would
partly offset their anxiety about his independence from
them. They also seemed to put less pressure on Hassan, and
Mr Khan made some preliminary arrangements for him to
work in the same factory as he did. They were perhaps a
little relieved that he was likely to feel more at home with
his parents than Farrukh who would move, certainly some
of the time, in a very different world.

The intervention of the Child Care Officer could not
remove the tension between these parents and their children but it did make it more manageable. It also helped to
build a bridge between the family and the people concerned
with their children and to establish a number of authority
figures in a more friendly light. A great deal of bad feeling
and a number of misunderstandings were avoided as the
family felt that their position was respected and understood, even if not always agreed with. As a result, they felt
more able to make helpful contacts with other English
people.

Social workers cannot change the educational environment of the children with whom they are concerned, but
their agencies may be able to contribute to the special
help the Plowden Committee recommended for schools in
educational priority areas. For example, they may be able
to sponsor special holiday or after-school play schemes.
It may also be important for some social workers to have
special responsibility for liaison with the teachers and
parents in certain schools. These are services from which
all children, both white and coloured, could benefit.

Those who are concerned about the implications for race
relations in Britain of the growth of a poorly educated and
frustrated coloured minority need to be specially aware of

the educational problems of coloured school children. The school is a microcosm of the larger society. Its problems, and the policies designed to meet them, reflect the attitudes and priorities of society and determine its future. For no group is this more true than for immigrants and their children.

Immigrants and employment

Perhaps the most important factor shaping the future of immigrants and their descendants in Britain is the extent to which they are able to find employment commensurate with their abilities. The low wages and financial insecurity that accompany poor employment opportunities prevent immigrants from moving from the very areas which provide them and their children with the fewest chances of improving their economic and social position. All too easily the immigrant can find himself entangled in a vicious circle of poor employment, low wages, and inadequate housing and other facilities.

When they first arrive in Britain, immigrants, anxious to establish themselves and pay off debts accumulated during their immigration, are willing to take any work available, including some of the hardest jobs in the most ill-equipped industries, employment in public services such as transport, domestic and labouring jobs in hospitals, and some of the most menial catering work. Some, indeed, may know that for various reasons, including their own lack of skills and training, it is unlikely that they will be able to improve their situation greatly during their working lives, although many of them rightly expect the promotion and seniority that normally accompany long service. The attitude of their children will be different, especially if they have received all their education here and they will expect employment opportunities commensurate with their abilities. In addition, it should be remembered that many immigrants now coming to work in Britain, particularly since 1965, are well-qualified people who expect to find skilled or professional employment.

Given this background of skills and expectations, it is probably not surprising that the 1961 and 1966 censuses show that, on the whole, coloured immigrants are grossly over represented in the lowest socio-economic groups. There are some variations between the different groups and in different parts of the UK, and some anomalies which show, for example, that West Indian women appear to be welcomed as nurses but not as clerical or administrative workers.

Partly because no separate records of the employment of the children of immigrants are kept, and partly because of the large number of new immigrants in Britain in the last ten years, the census cannot yet show whether immigrants from the New Commonwealth are achieving, or are likely to achieve, employment similar to that of other immigrant groups, such as the Irish, and ultimately to that of the rest of the population. A number of factors make it unlikely that they will be able to do this. The limited life chances of many coloured immigrants and their families, which prevent them from realizing their full potential, will effectively exclude them from some of the employment requiring qualified workers. Perhaps even more serious is the extent of the discrimination against coloured people which drastically limits the number and type of jobs available to them. In particular, some jobs involving contact with the public, including work in banking, insurance, and some shop work, are virtually closed to coloured immigrants. Careers officers also say that it is hard to obtain apprenticeships and clerical work for coloured school leavers, particularly those within the middle range of ability. In general, it takes longer to find coloured school leavers suitable employment and very often the jobs they obtain are not those to which they had aspired. A combination of poor educational attainment, the discriminatory practices of employers, and sometimes the tendency of careers officers and others to see coloured school leavers as capable only of unskilled and routine work, can result in young coloured people being placed in low status work providing few opportunities. So serious are the implications of these poor employment opportunities that the Select Committee set up by the government to study race relations and immigration looked first at the problems of coloured school leavers. Their report, which makes largely gloomy reading, was published in 1969.

Various studies have revealed substantial discrimination against coloured employees seeking promotion or further training. Even the terms and conditions of work for coloured employees may be inferior to those for white employees. They may have to accept the least convenient shifts and have few opportunities for working overtime. The level of this discrimination makes it likely that even those who have had all their education in Britain and are well qualified may find their colour a barrier in employment. We do not yet know how successful the 1968 Race Relations Act will be in reducing this discrimination, partly because legal machinery provides a cumbersome method of preserving individual rights. Although we must be cautious in making comparisons between the United States and Britain, it is worth taking note of the findings of the National Advisory Commission on Civil Disorders (1968) which studied the background to the recent riots in American cities:

> The typical rioter was a teenager or young adult, a life-long resident of the city in which he rioted, a high school drop-out; he was, nevertheless, somewhat better educated than his Negro neighbour and was usually under-employed or employed in a menial job. He was proud of his race, extremely hostile to whites and middle-class Negroes, and, although informed about politics, highly distrustful of the political system (p. 7).

Social workers cannot alter the over-all employment situation of immigrants, but they must be aware of the frustrations and bitterness which many immigrants feel when faced not only with their own poor employment but also that of their children. Apart from affecting a family's economic position, a vicious circle of poor employment opportunities, particularly if they seem to result from discrimination on the part of employers, can strain the relationships within a family. Great pressure may be brought to bear on children to get the kind of qualifications which will ensure them better jobs than their parents, and immigrants may also be reluctant for themselves or their children to give up an unsatisfactory job lest it should be impossible to find another. It may be useful for a social worker to help the members of a family to discuss amongst themselves the fears, hopes, and disappointments which influence their actions because, when these are not understood or acknowledged, misunderstanding and bitterness can persist.

Some people see the ambitions of many immigrant parents for their children as unrealistic and this has been discussed in the previous section. In their work with coloured people, social workers have to be very honest with themselves in their assessment of children's abilities and opportunities. They will know some parents, both immigrant and native, who have invested all their frustrated hopes and ambitions in their children who, for various reasons, are unequal to them. There are times when it is right for social workers to help people to come to terms with their limited abilities and the employment opportunities open to them, and to see their individual worth in terms other than just the job they are able to do. Furthermore, to attempt to modify parental ambitions or to discourage young coloured people from seeking certain kinds of work may well save from rebuffs and disappointment. On the other hand, in doing this social workers may be subscribing quite unthinkingly to the general view that coloured people are only suitable for certain kinds of work; they may also be helping to stultify the ambition, the willingness to work hard and endure hardship which are some of the most precious assets of immigrant families. In many cases it may well be better for social workers to do everything in their power to help young coloured people to obtain the kind of work they want, even if this means delays and frustrations. These efforts could include discussions with employers, teachers, and careers officers, accompanying young applicants to the places of employment and sometimes even to their interviews, and a willingness to bear with their disappointments. Such help is particularly important for young coloured people who are unlikely to find employment in firms run by people of their own national origin. While Indians and Cypriots. have been successful in establishing small businesses and other entrepreneurial activities which offer employment to people of a similar national background, such opportunities are not available to most other immigrant groups.

When social workers are aware of the discriminatory practices of employers, they should discuss these with officers of the Race Relations Board.

Residential social workers are faced with a similar dilemma. Children in residential care are frequently protected from the harsh realities of life outside. In particular, coloured children may be unprepared for the discrimination they may meet in their search for employment. It will be especially hard for them to cope with this without the support of their own families. Although residential workers want to ease the entry of children in their care into the world of employment, they are often reluctant to discuss with them problems associated with colour. Sometimes they feel that this will imply discrimination on their part; sometimes they wish to avoid unpleasant issues and may feel that such discussions could lead children to exaggerate or look for difficulties that are not there; sometimes they believe that it is wrong to say anything to children which could imply their inferior status or limited opportunities.

What seems most important for children in residential care is that they should be able to share their problems as they arise with those who care for them, and that no subjects should be seen as taboo. In particular, this implies special help and support for adolescent children, especially when they are looking for jobs. It may be that coloured children at this time need extra encouragement and help to find employment and lodgings. We should bear in mind Erikson's (1965) words: 'ego identity gains real strength only from the whole hearted and consistent recognition of real accomplishment i.e. of achievement that has meaning in the culture' (p. 228).

It is in the search for employment that social workers must be particularly aware of both the long- and short-term needs of coloured immigrants; their prosperity and security, as well as that of the rest of the community, are bound up with the work they are able to do.

Immigrants and the police

The decaying centres of large towns are also the areas where the highest crime rates are to be found and therefore, necessarily, the focus of much police activity. Crime in this context is not the highly organized work of professional criminals playing for high stakes; most typically it means petty theft, drunkenness, prostitution, and minor violence resulting from disputes between landlords and tenants and the friction which is inevitable amongst families when large numbers of people are crowded together in totally inadequate accommodation.

In a study of a Birmingham police division, Lambert (1970) has shown (as have several other criminologists) that, difficult though it is to make satisfactory comparisons between the crime rates of different national or ethnic groups, coloured immigrants and their children are very much less involved than their white neighbours with the extensive criminal activities which are part of their immediate environment. Nevertheless, evidence from other countries, particularly the USA, suggests that if the legitimate aspirations of second-generation immigrants are frustrated and there is no escape from the poorest neighbourhoods and most menial employment, the crime rate amongst them will increase very substantially to match, or even exceed, that of individuals from long established families. Crime may then become associated with the activities of a coloured minority rather than being seen as the inevitable consequence of general deprivation and urban decay.

Lambert detects the beginnings of this association among some police working in the inner city, despite the fact that all the evidence belies it. Lack of everyday contact with coloured people, except in the course of investigating crime, and ignorance about their cultural background and life style in Britain, lead to the possibility of stereotyping coloured people as deviant. Their obvious visibility also makes it easier for them to be chosen as the subjects of police enquiries. Problems of communication are increased when immigrants' perception and expectations of the British police are shaped by their experience of police forces in their native countries where corruption and violence may be common. Opportunities for mutual recrimination multiply when fear or ignorance prompt unnecessarily aggressive or devious responses. If this is the context of the relationship between immigrants and the police, it is not surprising that many coloured people complain of police harassment and, like their white neighbours, are frequently not satisfied that their complaints are dealt with impartially. John (1970), one of the contributors to a revealing study published by the Runnymede Trust, describes most vividly mounting hostility between the police and young coloured people living in a particularly poor district. He also perceptively discusses the reasons for deteriorating relationships.

These tensions are only the most extreme example of

the problems which arise between the police and deprived communities when the ambiguities of the police role are not resolved. Not only are the police required to pursue a relentless war against crime, which inevitably means a concentration of their detective activities in some of the poorest urban areas, they are also expected to contribute to the prevention of crime and the maintenance of law and order by fostering good relationships with the public, especially those most likely to be alienated from them. The deprivation and the neglect experienced by the inhabitants of these neighbourhoods, combined with the social distance between them and the police, create formidable barriers to these relationships. In Lambert's words, 'the police, as symbols of authority in society are seen as upholders not only of the law and order of society's aspirations but also of the lawlessness and injustice of society in action' (p. xxi). To a large extent, the police, as the most available and tangible figures of authority, bear the brunt of the consequences of the negligence and apparent indifference of society towards its poorest members.

Just as the priorities of the police reflect the priorities of a society which is more anxious about a rising crime rate than the social conditions of which it is a product, so do the attitudes of coloured people towards the police reveal the possibility of a growing sense of alienation of the urban poor from those who have power over them, that is, the civil servants, politicians, and social workers; and yet it is on these people that they are, of necessity, heavily dependent. The police are not alone in their need to explore ways of maintaining communication with, and the confidence of, some of the most needy and vulnerable people in our society.

Some implications for social work

This catalogue of deprivations, which can cripple the inhabitants of the poorest urban areas, makes it tempting

57

for social workers to believe that there is nothing social work departments, let alone individual social workers, can do to alleviate the more general problems which pervade these neighbourhoods. Although they spend much of their time working with families in these districts, they are often pessimistic about the outcome of their activities, seeing their work frequently as a 'patching up' process, the delaying of crises, or the provision of some short-term relief for acute and chronic difficulties. They are often aware that only satisfactory housing will substantially relieve the problems of many families; and like many other people, they may believe that only the wholesale redevelopment of some areas will bring an end to their degradation and squalor, although they know that sometimes such programmes exchange old problems for new ones.

These frustrations have spurred many social workers to reassess their aims and methods of work. Realizing that whatever long-term plans may exist for them, these central urban areas will be the environment in which many families will live for several years, they are finding it important to focus on their strengths, to think of ways in which existing resources can be directed towards them, and to devise special help for their peculiar problems. These efforts are intended to help all their inhabitants, of whom immigrants are some of the more vulnerable.

1 *The accessibility of social services* There is evidence that many people living in the poorest districts do not ask for help that is available, sometimes because they do not know it exists and sometimes because they believe that those who have authority to give it are remote from, and unsympathetic to, their world. While some social work departments have established branch offices in new housing estates, it is too often assumed that those who live in the older, more central areas can easily find their way to the social work agencies. What is neglected is the fact that many of those living in these areas are newcomers, quite

unfamiliar with the provisions of the Welfare State and the workings of bureaucracy. In some cases, too, the depression and apathy which grip these twilight zones lead many people to believe that there is little they can do to improve their conditions and that there is no point in asking for help since they will probably be ignored. In such circumstances it is important for a social work department to have a branch in these neighbourhoods which will be more accessible and familiar than a large central department. In many cases these offices need to be served not only by caseworkers and other officials of the local authority department, but also by community workers. There are many advantages to this concentration of interest and resources. Not least, it provides a means whereby social workers can feel an identification with certain areas and become more familiar with their strengths and weaknesses.

2 *The need for information* The few communal institutions in the areas in which many immigrants live and the immigrants' dependence on a small family network, which can provide far less support than they could expect in their home countries, mean a greater reliance on social services, the functions or even the existence of which may be only dimly perceived. Although by no means unique in this respect, immigrants are amongst those most likely to be confused about their rights and obligations and overwhelmed by bureaucratic machinery. Burney (1967), for example, found that many immigrants were quite unaware that they might be eligible for a council house and few knew how to apply for one. They did not realize that their changes of address should be reported to welfare departments and that failure to do this or to renew their application for council housing could mean their being dropped from a waiting list. They were also unaware of house mortgage facilities provided by many local authorities which could do much to ease their housing problems.

Many immigrants are also quite bemused by the law and

regulations affecting the relationship between landlord and tenant and quite unable, without assistance, to get adequate legal advice or redress. Some immigrants, too, are not clear about the protection given by the Race Relations Act and, for various reasons, may be unwilling to report cases of discrimination, with the result that many people feel that it is safe to continue behaving in a discriminatory way towards coloured people. Immigrants may also be unaware of the regulations concerning the daily minding of children and, partly as a result of this, may unwittingly arrange for their children to be cared for in very unsatisfactory surroundings. Ignorance of these regulations may also mean that some immigrant women who agree to look after other people's children may take in more children than they can adequately care for given their limited accommodation and facilities.

It is not suggested that better information about existing services and more adequate access to legal and administrative machinery would necessarily solve the problems of those who live in the poorest areas, but their absence means that existing services are not used by the very people who need them most. And this lack of information is a two-way process because if services are not requested by those who need them, those who provide them will never learn the extent of un-met need. Bennington (1970) has also suggested that in areas where some redevelopment is already going on, with the consequent confusion about rehousing, demolition, and building programmes, the need for clear information about these plans and the chance for some consultation about them is valued more highly than an increase or improvement in personal social services. Burney (1967) has described vividly the fate of families, many of whom are immigrants, who move from house to house, unaware of the implications of redevelopment plans and the chance of rehousing by the local authority and always just 'one step ahead of the bulldozer' in their desperate struggle to secure a roof over their heads. Apart from their intrinsic value, efforts to provide information and opportunities to participate in the making of decisions about matters of acute personal importance may reduce the call on social services, by relieving some of the stress and anxiety inherent in a situation in which it is impossible to plan ahead with security.

The advertising of social services is surrounded by controversy and confusion about the extent of their universality and the rights and duties of those who need their help. The Seebohm Report (1968) pointed to the need to make services more widely known, and special efforts will be necessary to reach immigrants. For example, notices and leaflets in the appropriate languages could be displayed in shops owned or used extensively by immigrants, in their places of worship, and in their newspapers. Approaches could also be made to immigrant organizations. Some of this work is already done by Citizen's Advice Bureaux, but the reorganization of social work departments and concentration of resources provide an excellent opportunity for local authorities to make their services known and to sponsor special help for those new problems which may emerge.

An example of social work in a deprived neighbourhood

This account of the work of a small group of social workers illustrates some of the problems already described and ways in which they could be approached.

These social workers, representing different agencies, had been given the use of an old shop as a base for their activities in an area scheduled for redevelopment where some demolition work had already started. In the course of informal discussion, they realized that nearly all of them spent a large part of their time with families who lived in one street in six houses given over to multi-occupation. These houses were in bad repair, and their entrances and stairs depressing and dingy; but the rooms occupied by the families, although overcrowded, were almost uniformly bright and cheerful and bore witness to efforts to make the best of a poor environment.

In all, twenty-four families had needed help of some kind. Some of the social workers and health visitors were concerned about the welfare of children, many of whom had been in care for short periods during their mothers' confinements. The probation officers were aware of a number of neighbours' quarrels which had been referred to them but about which they felt they could do very little. They also knew that several people had serious legal problems concerned with landlord-tenant relationships and that some landlords had been prosecuted for overcrowding. The mental welfare officers were concerned with a number of women who had spent short periods in psychiatric hospitals and their case notes indicated that their breakdowns had been associated with stress arising from housing problems. Most of the social workers were also concerned about the care of young children whose mothers went out to work; they were also aware of potential conflict between parents and adolescent children living at very close quarters. The social workers were concerned that they usually came to hear of problems only when they had reached the point of crisis, often requiring drastic action. Those families who had had quite recent contact with a social worker only rarely asked for any further help, even when this was needed quite urgently. This lack of communication did not seem to arise from a reluctance to accept help or hostility to social workers once they had become involved with a family, but rather with confusion or vagueness about the availability of services. Those people who were referred elsewhere after approaching a social worker already known to them about a new problem outside his province, rarely made any attempt to follow up introductions made on the assumption that people would find it fairly easy to make themselves and their problems known to strange people who seemed remote from their environment. It was also well known that these twenty-four families frequently did not fill in or return the various forms which are a necessary part of bureaucracy. This failure did not just seem to be associated with an inability to understand the most complicated forms; the piles of uncollected dusty letters and circulars bearing an official stamp which are a feature of the hallways of so many houses of this kind, indicated a lack of awareness or concern about the importance of such communications.

After making a rough analysis of these cases, the social workers discovered that all the families were immigrants in that they had arrived in the city less than three years previously. Some were Irish or Scottish, but the majority were from the New Commonwealth. Of these, the largest number were West Indian, although there were several Pakistani families. In addition, four of the landlords were known to be Pakistanis, one a West Indian, and the remaining two English.

Most of their problems were associated either with housing and friction between tenants or landlord and tenants, or with difficulties over the care and upbringing of children. Clearly the partial solving of problems which had already reached crisis point, the reluctance to ask for help before this, and the division of responsibility amongst several social workers, were unsatisfactory.

The social workers thought that little would be achieved merely by circulating written information about their presence in the district and the services they could offer. They decided, therefore, to visit all the families in these houses personally and that one of them should be responsible for all the visits to one house. They realized that to be effective, these visits should aim at more than just introducing the social worker and providing information of a general nature about available services, and they decided to offer some particular information about the redevelopment plans in the immediate area, believing that this would be a source of concern for nearly all the families. In the course of discussion about these plans and their implications for the families, they hoped to learn something of their other difficulties. Their primary aim, however, was to establish themselves as people with access to useful information, whose role was to offer some help of their own initiative rather than being available only in times of crisis.

The social workers were initially uncertain about the value of these preliminary visits. Although they found people concerned about the local redevelopment proposals and also discovered that there was practically no contact between the families living in the same house, there were no immediate requests for any specific help. However, the demolition of some houses in the same street started a trickle of anxious enquiries about rehousing and the social worker who had paid the initial visit to each house made himself responsible for providing information about council policies. Several West Indians either put their names down or renewed their applications for council housing, and some Pakistani families, interested in house purchase, were told of the local authority mortgage schemes and helped to apply for them. They had originally intended to borrow money privately at very high rates of interest. In the course of looking for houses, some coloured families were told by an agent that all the houses on a new estate had been sold. The social workers knew this was not so and contacted the local conciliation officer from the Race Relations Board and asked him if he would discuss with the agent the sale of houses to coloured people.

During the course of all these negotiations, several families mentioned problems with their landlords over rent and repairs. It was also clear that some landlords turned a blind eye to overcrowding resulting from families accommodating friends and relatives and were fairly tolerant over rent arrears. The rents would certainly have been reduced if referred to the rent tribunal, but most of the families did not seem eager to do this and the social workers decided to try to discuss some of the tenants' problems with the landlords themselves. Those whom they did manage to see were angry and confused about their obligations as landlords. They were having to pay off short-term mortgages at high interest rates, could not obtain grants for improving their property, and were very uncertain or dissatisfied about the compensation they would eventually receive from the local authority. The landlords who had been prosecuted for overcrowding or failing to do necessary repairs, were incensed and bewildered by regulations which, on the one hand, demanded reasonable rents and outlay on improvement and, on the other, fixed the number of tenants allowed. Abiding by these regulations would make it impossible for some of them to cover their basic expenses, let alone undertake substantial improvements. They also pointed out, quite rightly, that practically no other landlords were willing to take families with young children, particularly coloured families, and that they were, therefore, offering an essential service. The social workers thought that even though some landlords exaggerated their difficulties, there was some justice to their complaints; and however unsatisfactory the general position, given the appalling shortage of housing, the interests of these tenants and landlords were not in total conflict. They offered the landlords some advice about their legal position and discussed the implications of the redevelopment proposals. At the same time they tried to persuade them to carry out essential repairs. In this they were not very successful, and a good deal of tension remained between the landlords and their tenants although it did not break into open conflict, partly because each side understood something of the other's position and recognized some mutual interests.

In taking this rather passive role, the social workers realized that they could be seen as colluding with an unsatisfactory state of affairs. Some people might have preferred to take a firmer stand and persuade the tenants to get their rents reduced. The social workers, however, were reluctant to put too much pressure on people to do something which might not be in their long-term interests, if, for example, it led ultimately to their eviction. Had the landlords indulged in threatening or aggressive behaviour they might have decided to act differently, but as it was, they saw themselves caught in a dilemma involving families with a greet need for accommodation, and relatively easy-going, accepting landlords willing to provide this at a price which, although high, did not necessarily mean they were making great profits. This dilemma they tried to explain to the Health and Housing Departments whose activities seemed to be inconsistent in that they both tried to limit the operations of some landlords who provided much needed accommodation, and yet failed to make alternative accommodation available.

The social workers were also concerned that one of the single mothers appeared to be minding the children of some of her neighbours in very unsatisfactory crowded conditions. She was not a registered daily minder and, although a capable and loving person, was quite unable to look after the children properly in one room. While being most concerned about these children's welfare, the social workers were reluctant to curtail the activities of someone who was providing an essential service for some mothers who had to work. They knew quite well that none of their children would be able to get places in nursery schools and that the fees of registered daily minders, even if they could be found, would be too high. After prolonged negotiations with the Children's and Health Departments it was agreed that a small 'nursery' could be established in a recently vacated flat in the basement of one of the houses. The Children's Department provided money for the rent and also for some essential repairs and decoration which were mostly carried out by the families using the nursery. This was important in itself as it was the first co-operative activity amongst the tenants. The original daily minder continued to care for the children although the local branch of the pre-school playgroups association provided her with a regular helper. The Health Visitor also carefully supervised the whole project.

The establishment of this nursery marked the beginning of a number of small co-operative projects amongst some of the tenants. The fathers were put in touch with a community worker who was trying to start an adventure playground and needed some helpers. One tenant, who delivered paraffin to the houses in the area, offered to inspect and repair oil stoves on the spot at very reduced rates for his regular customers. An elderly crippled lady who had occupied a small rent-controlled flat for a long time and who had been angered, and even frightened, by the arrival of these immigrant families, offered, after long discussions with one of the social workers, to teach sewing to four very isolated Pakistani girls whose parents never let them leave their flat after they returned from school. In return, their parents offered to pay for these lessons, but eventually it was agreed that it would be more helpful if they did some shopping and odd jobs for the old lady.

In the course of all these activities, the social workers found they were being consulted about a number of family difficulties with which they were able to give some help, partly because they were now involved before these problems had reached boiling-point, but also because they were now seen as genuinely helpful people who could be trusted to work in the interests of the families concerned.

All these projects were extremely time-consuming and it is difficult to assess their results accurately. In preventive terms, it is likely that much was achieved: some families had hopes of rehousing either through the local authority or by house purchase; some children received more adequate daily care; perhaps most important of all, the families began to feel less isolated and neglected and to see themselves as having some control over their present and future circumstances. Partly as a result of this, some of the more active tenants were prepared to involve themselves in a number of co-operative activities in the district and were helped to do this by a community worker. The social workers also noticed a marked reduction of tension amongst the families and far fewer overt signs of racial antagonism. Although there were still quarrels between neighbours and an obvious status hierarchy amongst the different racial groups, there was also a recognition of common problems and some co-operative activity. The number of direct requests for social work help increased, but the social workers felt that since they were being involved before problems became unmanageable, they were more effective in their work than they had been previously.

Although the majority of these families remained grossly underprivileged, some of their most immediate problems were relieved in valuable and tangible ways and they were more able to seek out other available help. This was achieved largely by the activities of social workers, who were nearly all caseworkers and who were prepared to think carefully about the aims and methods of their work and co-operate closely in directing their energies towards solving some of the urgent day-to-day problems which were of the greatest concern to the families and with which they would otherwise have been able to get very little help.

Community work

It is now widely accepted that community workers have a substantial contribution to make in deprived areas although their different methods of work and their success are only beginning to be evaluated. It is only possible here to outline briefly some of their activities, particularly as they concern immigrants.

Some community workers see the presence of immigrants in these neighbourhoods as representing potentially one of their greatest untapped strengths. Although it has been assumed that most of those who live in slums or twilight zones wish to leave them, some recent studies have shown that at least a substantial minority would like to stay, particularly if local amenities were improved. They include the older residents who have put down roots in an area and see little for themselves elsewhere, as well as many immigrants who either like the security of a neighbourhood where a number of their relatives or fellow countrymen live or who, as recent owner-occupiers, would like to improve their property and its immediate environment. Many immigrants are ambitious people, who have by their migration demonstrated their ability to plan ahead and their willingness to delay seeking immediate reward for their efforts. They do not share the hopelessness and apathy of those whose life experience has taught them there is little they can do to alter their circumstances. The immigrants who have recovered from the immediate stresses of migration have, therefore, the potential, perhaps with the encouragement of a community worker, to initiate or participate in a number of activities helpful to the district in which they live. However, these activities may also be the source of tension as they can inspire envy, as well as hope, amongst other local people.

Ideally, most community workers, and those who employ them, hope that in their efforts to help people to identify and make known their needs and to press for the creation or improvement of some services, the many disparate groups in the poorest areas will become aware of their common problems and co-operate with each other in solving them. Rex and Moore (1967) have described how the Sparkbrook Association made up of a number of people with very diverse backgrounds and interests managed to unite their efforts to improve certain amenities, for example by arranging that a street should be given a face lift. They were also able to draw attention to the poor facilities in Sparkbrook and get the local authority to provide or sponsor some services such as an adventure playground. One of the chief successes of the Association was to provide people with an avenue to express their grievances and to attempt to do something about them, so preventing a retreat into a racialist response which identified the existence of problems with the presence of immigrants. No longer was there such low morale with its resulting apathy and bitterness. This is no mean achievement and undoubtedly these successes of local community organizations are important to all those who belong to them and who are affected by their efforts.

There are, however, some people who are doubtful about the possibility, and indeed the use, of such co-operation which they see only as a veneer, sometimes imposed by well-meaning officials, over underlying and frequently serious tensions. For example, contributors to a Runnymede Trust publication (1970) believe that although in areas where there is already considerable social fragmentation, immigrants and natives need to discover a community of interests and aspirations, they will only be able to do this meaningfully and effectively from the basis of their own organizations, whose primary aims may be the pursuit of the apparently exclusive interests of their members. They accept both the necessity for, and value of, social and political associations which reflect the experience and culture of immigrants and natives, and believe that these distinct communities must be recognized. At least initially, only limited co-operation between them will be possible. 'Integration does not exist: it may be an ultimate goal or policy, it should not determine the style of action' (p. 49).

Two important principles underlie this understanding of community needs and the ways in which they can be met. In the first place, it is assumed that ordinary members of the public should be involved in planning and decision-making about matters which intimately affect their lives. Although this kind of participation is now a familiar theme in politics and social philosophy, it is more usually an ideal than an effective policy. Some people believe that it is only possible if individuals organize themselves into groups which they believe represent their own interests and which give them security, confidence, and some power both to negotiate with other interest groups and to provide their own self-help schemes. Although such groups may make many mistakes and political blunders, they can offer people the dignity of feeling that they have some control over their own lives.

The second assumption is that since these different groups will not always see themselves, sometimes quite inaccurately, as sharing the same problems requiring the same solutions, they are more likely initially to compete than to co-operate with each other. Whether these tensions break into open conflict depends partly on their ideals and partly on the balance of power between the groups. Community workers have a contribution to make in helping them negotiate with each other and advising them about appropriate strategies.

Considerable anxiety is often expressed about the formation of associations, perhaps organized on a national or ethnic basis, which could define problems in racial terms. Undoubtedly their activities involve some risk, but the community workers who accept these principles believe that it is more important to work within the context of existing tensions than to ignore them. Depending on the ways in which they are expressed, they see these tensions as potentially constructive. They think it important to use and encourage existing 'natural' self-interest groups, believing the only alternative, except for the most educated and politically sophisticated, to be self-contempt, apathy, and alienation.

Both these approaches to community work, the one

highlighting consensus, and the other, conflict between groups, have a contribution to make; decisions about which is the most appropriate must take into account the needs of the areas and individuals concerned. But the potential of community work programmes must not be exaggerated. They may be able to draw attention to areas of deprivation and do something to improve existing facilities. They may help some individuals with particular problems and ensure chances of communication between ordinary people and those who make decisions about their future. They may encourage associations which give their members confidence and an identity. However, they cannot on their own do much to change the general pattern of underprivilege in an area and it is probable that large numbers of people will be little affected by their activities. Hill and Issacharoff (1971) have shown how community relations committees, established to promote multi-racial harmony, and partly supported by funds from central government, are unlikely to be effective in improving the general underprivileged of immigrants for a variety of reasons, including limited resources, confusion about aims, an inevitable pressure on them to compromise, often unhelpfully, with more powerful white organizations, and the inconsistent behaviour of the government in the field of race relations. They are more successful in promoting smaller but valuable activities such as playgroups and information services. Those community work projects which aim to work on a less official basis, with a number of different interest groups, often find their activities limited by internal dissensions which are sometimes an inevitable preliminary to the identification of common concerns and strategies. Various evaluations of community work in the USA have come to similar conclusions. Details of some of these studies are given in the suggestions for further reading.

Community work is now fashionable, but social workers need to be aware of its limitations as well as its advantages lest they should give the misleading impression that it can solve gross problems of deprivation.

Positive discrimination

'... to achieve equality, resources must be unevenly distributed to counterbalance the gross inequalities which already exist' (Seebohm Report, 1968, p. 150).

Perhaps the most important principle which social workers and local authorities should adopt in their work in the poorest areas is that they need special attention and extra resources if their standard of living is to improve. This principle is already being put into effect in some education priority areas, community development projects, and the urban aid programme. These schemes do not have personalized targets of help, but aim to give extra resources to particular neighbourhoods or age groups within them. Social workers would accept this general principle as important, but they may also think that some groups need special attention. The serious difficulties faced by many immigrants and the grave consequences of their entrapment in a vicious circle of underprivilege, possibly resulting in the association of colour with poverty now so familiar in the USA, may call for this extra help. Such decisions have to be made with care and judgment, as well as courage. This is the price of helping those with the greatest needs.

4

The strains of migration

I shall touch upon broken homes, interruptions of family life, separation from known surroundings, the becoming a foreigner and ceasing to belong. These are the aspects of alienation; and seen from the perspective of the individual received rather than the receiving society, the history of immigration is a history of alienation and its consequences (Handlin, 1953, p. 41).

The process of migration means both fulfilment and problems for many individuals and families. Many of these problems have been experienced by all those who uproot themselves from their native countries and attempt to settle in a strange land. However, some special difficulties await immigrants whose customs and cultural traditions are very different from those of the country of immigration.

Some general problems

1 *Financial difficulties* Although most immigrants can expect to earn far more than would be possible in their native countries, many of them face severe financial difficulties, especially in the first years after their arrival. The previous section has shown that immigrants are frequently concentrated in the industries which offer the lowest wages and that they often have to pay out large sums for housing. Although immigrants are usually young and there-

fore at the height of their earning power, the young families which characterize this age group involve heavy expenditure. Some studies have shown that the earnings and household incomes of immigrants are generally lower than those of the whole population and that there is particular hardship in households consisting of several persons. Apart from those difficulties common to all low-wage earners with young families, immigrants also face extra demands on their financial resources. Their migration expenses are heavy and frequently involve family debt. In addition, since it is usually impossible for a whole family to emigrate together, many immigrants are saving hard for the fares for the rest of their family. These re-unions can also involve heavy expenditure over and above providing extra accommodation. Clothing suitable for a cold climate has to be bought, and frequently quite large sums must be spent to equip children for their new schools. Providing basic items of household equipment, such as heaters and cooking utensils, can also be expensive. Possibly one of the biggest claims on immigrants' incomes is the provision of support for family members who remain in the native countries. These include children who may expect one day to be reunited with their parents, but who in the meantime are cared for by other relatives, and older family members who may be completely dependent for their keep on their relatives living in Britain. Immigrants also are anxious to save large sums either to provide for their return to their native countries or to establish themselves here securely, perhaps by buying a house. In general, it is thought that immigrants save or send home up to a quarter of their income, compared with only 5 per cent of income saved by the British population as a whole.

Apart from these very severe financial demands, which often mean that immigrants are living at or below subsistence level and spending little on food, some feel they must demonstrate to themselves and to others that they are making their way towards a more luxurious standard of living by possessing such articles as cocktail cabinets, radiograms, and television sets. These items are sometimes regarded by social workers and others as unnecessary extravagances; they should be seen rather as providing some immigrants with a feeling of achievement, of hopes and ambitions fulfilled, and, therefore, with some measure of security in a frequently hard and bleak existence.

We do not yet know how many immigrants fulfil their ambitions in terms of accumulating enough capital to establish themselves securely in Britain or to return to buy land or a business in their native countries. What is clear is that the heavy demands on their income, combined with many other practical problems, involve constant strain and anxiety. This means that many immigrant families believe they must exploit their total wage-earning power even if this causes serious practical problems in the care of their children. It can also mean that parents want their wage-earning children to contribute all or the major part of their wages to the family budget. It is quite possible that the thrift practised by immigrants and their great interest in establishing themselves materially will not be viewed sympathetically by their children or, indeed, by the many people for whom expenditure on entertainment and luxuries is more important than the accumulation of savings.

2 *Difficulties concerning immigration procedures* Bagley (1969) has produced some evidence that uncertainties about the complicated immigration laws and procedures are a cause of major anxiety in immigrant families. Administrative and other delays may mean that children pass the legal age limit for admission to Britain to join their parents. Furthermore, the law can operate to divide families whom traditional obligations of kinship would unite. Inevitably, uncertainty about possible changes in immigration laws which may remove the right of dependants to

enter Britain, is a nagging source of worry and insecurity. In its enquiry into the control of Commonwealth immigration, the Select Committee on Race Relations and Immigration (1969-70), discovered most disturbing evidence of unnecessary hardship and delays experienced by immigrants in Britain and potential immigrants in their native countries in their attempts to gain the necessary permission for entry to Britain. This Committee's report describes most vividly the extraordinary persistence and ability needed by prospective migrants in their attempts to obtain legally obligatory entry vouchers in their native countries. It must be remembered that in this sphere the inefficiencies and injustices of bureaucracy, now to some extent countered by an appeals procedure, may mean that close relatives will be separated from each other for the rest of their lives. It is not surprising that a major concern for many families lies in their attempt to understand and comply with the regulations surrounding immigration from the Commonwealth.

3 *Homesickness and adjustment* The homesickness experienced by many immigrants can be acute. It is probably hard for anyone who has not travelled to a distant and unfamiliar country and been separated from most or all of his family to imagine the feelings of loss, fear, and isolation which can be part of an immigrant's daily life. Many will long for their relatives, uncertain of when they will be reunited. Letters, a difficult form of communication for some people, may be infrequent. For some years, there will probably be little hope of a holiday at home. In the absence of news, some immigrants will be extremely worried about their families and yet often powerless to find out how they are. Many, too, have good cause for anxiety. For example, some Asian families, in particular, take a risk in sending to Britain their young male members, the most likely to command the highest wages, because this usually means a reduction in the family's income until

money is sent home. Immigrants may, therefore, be anxious that their already poor dependants may be suffering even greater hardship. They may also be concerned that their farms or small businesses are being neglected in their absence.

Those immigrants who have to leave their children behind in the care of relatives will not only miss them but be anxious about their progress. Letters which complain of their bad behaviour or imply that relatives are no longer able or willing to care for them, can be a source of frantic worry for immigrant parents who for reasons of finance or lack of accommodation may be quite unable to bring their children to the UK.

These specific anxieties and feelings of homesickness are made more acute because of the unfamiliarity of most immigrants with the British way of life. Again, it is hard for most people to understand the great differences between the urban and rural life of the countries of emigration and that of the UK. The construction of buildings, the methods of transport, the shops and supermarkets, the planning of cities, and, perhaps above all, the weather, which forces people to stay inside their houses for most of the year in cramped conditions, are all unfamiliar and unwelcoming to most immigrants. These are the things which many immigrants who have lived here for some time find hard to describe and yet which contribute in no small way to their feelings of isolation. In addition, many immigrants are quite unfamiliar with the English language and are, therefore, unable to communicate properly with those whom they meet in the course of their daily lives. Apart from the obvious inconvenience, it can mean that immigrants feel they are never able to relax. They are constantly anxious that they will not be able to make themselves understood, even in the minor but necessary transactions involved in shopping or travelling. Although on their arrival some immigrants may be sheltered by relatives, they are soon faced with formidable practical problems which would severely tax the ingenuity and patience of longstanding residents. Although the English have a reputation for rather passive tolerance, they do not actively welcome those whom they regard as strangers and their coolness may convey hostility or contempt to many immigrants, particularly to those who experience substantial discrimination. An immigrant who has lived here for two or three years sums up these feelings well:

> When I first arrived I felt I was floating through a way of life and situations I didn't understand. It was an uncomfortable feeling because it meant I didn't have any contact with anyone. People in shops and on buses looked at me strangely. I felt a fool; I couldn't even explain where I was going or what I wanted to buy. I didn't understand the small things people say to each other which make you feel at home. I felt pushed around, without any direction, in a crowd which was quite strange. Even now I get this feeling of detachment, of living in a limbo where neither you nor anyone else understands or cares what is going on. But at times, when I could bear to think and feel, I cared very much. I would get sudden sharp memories and images of people and places back home. They seemed bathed in a warm and glowing light. Perhaps they weren't quite real, but they hurt all the same. I would want to cry; I longed to be talked to; I felt a quite childish need to be fed and fussed over, to be someone again. When things were very bad, I would go to bed and surround myself with hot water bottles and blankets and close my eyes and try to shut out this alien, unfriendly world and slip back into memories and then oblivion. At times I could hardly move and spent two or three days in bed. I didn't want to eat, I didn't care about myself; I felt the kind of nothing that everyone outside seemed to think I was.

Social workers under pressure to try to solve a number of practical problems quickly are often unaware of the depth of the misery and loneliness which is not very far beneath the surface of many immigrants' lives. But it is this unhappiness, which often lies behind an immigrant's apathy and withdrawal from problems, which can puzzle some social workers. For a time anyway, some immigrants may feel quite unable to cope with ordinary everyday problems; they may be emotionally labile and seem quite childish. This is the kind of behaviour which is typical of those who have temporarily to regress because of shock or an accumulation of strain. Social workers realize that chronic feelings of depression and the need to regress can severely handicap a person in his daily life, but the very fact that many immigrants, by dint of persistence and determination, do cope so well can obscure their struggle and unhappiness and their need to think and talk about their life before coming to Britain.

Sometimes, in an attempt to escape from their hard and dreary lives, and in their need to believe in a better alternative to which they can return if they so wish, immigrants idealize their home country and their life before emigration. Occasionally, their memories or accounts of the comfort and ease of this life may be unrealistic; none the less, it is important that social workers be willing to listen to them, partly because they may be the only people to whom immigrants can talk in this way, and partly because some immigrants need to establish an image of themselves which they find more comfortable than the one which accompanies their hard and often menial existence in the UK. The acceptance of this image by a social worker is often a necessary beginning to the establishment of a relationship in which an immigrant may be helped, not only with his practical problems, but with the chronic loneliness and unhappiness which make it so tempting to escape from everyday life to the world of the imagination.

Some immigrants may be quite unable to think about themselves, their situation in their new country, and their life at home for fear that they will break down if they do so. Selvon (1956, p. 170), a West Indian novelist, describes this feeling well:

as if on the surface things didn't look so bad, but when you go down a little, you bounce up a kind of misery and pathos and a frightening—what? He didn't know the right word, but he had the right feeling in his heart. As if the boys laughing, but they only laughing because they 'fraid to cry, they only laughing because to think so much about everything would be a big calamity—like how he here now, the thoughts so heavy like he unable to move his body.

When this sadness or depression is so great that it hinders people in their everyday lives and, especially when unspoken, threatens emotional health, social workers may need to help immigrants to air their grief and to have some experience of feeling their unhappiness more openly without being crippled by it. Lindemann (1965) has shown that those bereaved people who can mourn their loss freely, openly, and soon after a person's death are usually likely to make a better and quicker adjustment than those who cannot grieve in this way. The loss experienced by immigrants bears many similarities to that of the bereaved and in the period of crisis after their arrival, or when they are worried about absent relatives, immigrants may need intensive, although usually short-term help. Handlin (1953, p. 6) describes the experiences of migrants to America:

They lived in crisis because they were uprooted. In transportation, while the old roots were sundered, before the new were established, the immigrants lived in an extreme situation. The shock and the effects of the shock, persisted for many years; and their influence reached down to generations which themselves never paid the cost of crossing.

Some immigrants may expect these difficulties, but it is unlikely that they anticipate some of the problems of adjustment that many immigrants experience within their own families. Usually these are not immediately apparent but eventually, to a greater or lesser extent, most immigrants find their family relationships changed, and sometimes extremely painful, at a time when their comparative isolation from the rest of the population makes it urgent for them to find security and support within their own homes.

Changes in family structure and values

If I say this over and over again it is because it is what I feel most about this country—that here there is no room for affection in people's lives. This is true both of the English and of the Indians who come to live here— the Indians become like the English because they are working under the same conditions. Here no one takes thought for the other ... people are too busy making money for themselves to find time to love each other (Sharma, 1971, pp. 186-7).

Perhaps the most important and difficult change immigrants have to face in their families is the shift from a family unit composed of three or four generations, to which many relatives feel they belong and for which they bear some responsibility, to a much smaller one, perhaps consisting of only parents and children. These smaller families bear less responsibility for their relatives in the UK than they would do in their home countries. In return, they can expect less help from them than would have been the case before immigration. This change in family structure does not come about quickly, and migration can be sponsored and shared by whole family units. None the less, many immigrants eventually become aware that the longer they stay in Britain, the more individual family members are anxious to pursue their own interests in a way which would have been unheard of in their native countries.

We do not know how closely the structure of the families of immigrants will eventually resemble that of families long established in Britain. This will depend partly on the extent to which relatives are reunited, on the mobility of immigrants in their search for employment and a better standard of living, and on their wish and ability to retain customs and traditions of their native countries. There will also be variations amongst the different immigrant groups. However, it seems likely that those immigrants who come to Britain fairly late in life will need to look to the support of their relatives and will also recognize some responsibility for them. Decisions may be taken jointly and in the interests of the total family group rather than individual members.

Those who come to the UK at a young age, or the children of immigrants, may be far less happy with these mutual responsibilities and the concept of family life within a large group. They may wish for the independence which they think characterizes the way of life of those whose families have always lived in Britain, and they may call into question the values of their older relations. Some older immigrants are also likely to be aware that their beliefs and outlook on life do not necessarily fit easily with the competitive atmosphere and pursuit of individual interests which characterize advanced urban societies. Slowly, particularly if they have lived in a rural society, they may become aware that the criteria and conditions of success in the UK are quite different from those in their native countries. As Handlin (1953, pp. 5-6) describes it:

> The customary modes of behaviour were no longer adequate, for the problems of life were new and different. With old ties snapped, men faced the enormous compulsion of working out new relationships, new meaning to their lives, often under harsh and hostile circumstances.
> The responses of these folk could not be easy, auto-

matic, for emigration had stripped away the veneer that in most stable situations concealed the underlying nature of the social structure. Without the whole complex of institutions and social patterns which formerly guided their actions, the people became incapable of masking or evading decisions.

Under such circumstances, every act was crucial, the product of conscious weighing of alternatives, never simple conformity to an habitual pattern. No man could escape choices that involved, day after day, an evaluation of his goals, of the meaning of his existence and of the purpose of the social forms and institutions that surrounded him.

Many immigrants may experience that state of mind described by Merton as anomie. This implies a way of life characterized by a lack of certainty about norms and values; a feeling that the rules which formerly guided conduct have lost their force, savour, and legitimacy; and a lack of a social order in which people feel they can put their trust. However, it must not be forgotten that immigrants also share many of the values and aspirations of the urban societies to which they have come. They are ambitious and anxious to establish themselves materially and socially; they accept that this upward social mobility will probably require a willingness to move around the country and certainly to work hard. They differ in the extent of their commitment to these ideals, to which they frequently hold more strongly than most of the indigenous population. They may also be more willing to suffer the trials that accompany the pursuit of these goals. They differ, too, in their understanding of the terms of success, believing that it must involve the whole family rather than individual members. Only with the declining influence of the extended family do immigrants begin to feel confused about their relationships not only with the wider society but also within their immediate social group. 'The qualities that were desirable in the good peasant were not the most conducive to success in the transition. Neighbourliness, obedience, respect and status were valueless ... they succeeded who put aside the old preoccupations, pushed in and took care of themselves' (Handlin, 1953, p. 61).

Husbands and wives

The change in family structure, and in the values and outlook of individuals, can lead in some families to confusion and even bitterness. The relationship between husbands and wives may be strained, particularly in those Asian families where it is customary for women to lead a domestic and secluded life. Isolated from the support and companionship they could expect in their native countries, they frequently feel lonely and lost in the UK, aware that their lives are very different from those of many British women whose roles are not exclusively defined in terms of their bond to a husband and children. Sometimes the day-to-day tasks of running a home can seem overwhelming to a young inexperienced housewife who, in her native country, could have relied on the help and guidance of other female relatives. They may wonder and worry about the future of their children in Britain, and how far they will be willing to conform to their traditional pattern of life. Some may even doubt its continued relevance but need to discuss this with their families.

These women will need more contact with their husbands than would have been customary in their home countries. They may also find that they both want and need to take a greater part in the making of decisions concerning the family. In particular, it is likely that much will need to be discussed about the upbringing of children. Some Asian women find that they have to take the responsibilities which customarily fall to senior female family members far sooner than would be usual in their native countries. Inevitably there will be a few whose experience of a more passive role in family life has made them feel unequal to these responsibilities, while some may wish for greater independence than their husbands feel is right for them.

Even in those families where it has been customary for wives to work and to have some financial independence, both they and their husbands may be aware that most women in Britain have a relationship of some equality with their husbands, the extent of which is unfamiliar to some immigrants and which can be both a threat and an object of envy for them. How far men will be able to meet their wives' needs for support, companionship, and some independence, will depend partly on their view of their predicament and their feelings about possible changes in family life, and partly on the extent of financial and other strains which may leave them with little energy to cope with domestic problems. Men like Mr Khan, described in an earlier case history, for whom migration has meant a decline in social status and work in the most menial positions, may feel the need to exert themselves forcefully in their families and command the respect and authority which are denied them in their work and wider social relationships. They may do this just at the time when their wives and children are wanting a greater degree of sharing and informality within the family. In such circumstances, tension and clashes may be inevitable.

Although most families will manage these changes in relationship without too much difficulty, social workers need to remember that the smallness of the family units and the unaccustomed closeness and intensity of family relationships are likely to be bewildering, and some individuals may at first find their new family roles difficult and yearn for a return to the old ways. They may also be angry and resentful about the way of life in Britain which they see as responsible for some of the changes in their own families.

Parents and children

1 *Separation and reunion* Some of the greatest confusion and difficulties that families face as a result of their migration concern their children, and perhaps some of the hardest of these problems arise when parents are forced to leave their children in their native countries when emigrating to Britain. The extent of the difficulties connected with the separation of parents and children will depend on a number of factors including the age of the children at the time of separation, their relationship with their parents and the length of their separation from them, the quality of care they receive in their home countries, and the circumstances of their families when they are reunited with them.

Social workers are not alone in their concern about these separations which can undoubtedly cause some serious problems, but they may interpret them too much in the context of the pattern of family life with which they are most familiar. Unlike European children who are usually cared for almost entirely by their mothers, with some involvement on the part of the fathers, many children whose parents have emigrated to the UK have always been cared for by a fairly extensive family network involving grandparents, brothers and sisters, aunts and uncles. Their own parents may not always have been particularly involved in their care, having delegated it, for various reasons, to other relatives. The departure of these parents for Britain may not, therefore, be a tremendous loss and shock for their children, as they will continue to find most of the security they need with other relatives. But when the time comes for them to join their parents, and many children have very little time to prepare themselves for this, they will almost certainly grieve for the people who have cared for them all their lives, perhaps realizing that there is little chance they will ever see them again. It is as if these relatives were dead, and many children recently arrived in Britain experience a period of mourning which is not always recognized or understood by their families.

To the grief these children feel at separation from their relatives is added the shock of finding themselves in a totally unfamiliar country, living often in a confined space with people they hardly know or remember and, perhaps, in the company of younger brothers and sisters who seem to occupy most of the attention of their parents. The whole pattern of life of these children changes in a few hours and they may be confused about the responses required of them and quite without the comfort and support of those who have, until now, represented parental authority and love. For those children who were not part of such extended family networks and who experienced the dual separation from their mothers and then, perhaps, their grandmothers, the confusion and unhappiness may be even greater. Social workers need, therefore, to discover the pattern of a child's life before coming to Britain because there may be several factors contributing to a child's grief, loneliness, and possibly withdrawn or hostile behaviour apart from his initial separation from his mother. Whatever the circumstances of separation from close relatives, there is considerable evidence that it is an important contributing factor to the disturbed behaviour of immigrant children, especially those from the West Indies, whose domestic environment is often more insecure than that of Asian children.

It is easy to feel sympathy with children who have had this experience of a rapid transfer from a familiar to a strange world, and some social workers are angered by parents who appear not to understand the strains such a change places on their children. But these parents are also in a difficult position. Many have made great financial sacrifices to bring their children to this country and provide them with an adequate home and educational opportunities. They have worked and longed for the day when their family would be reunited. Encouraged by their relatives, their children too may have lived in anticipation of the day when they would be sent for by their parents. It can be a bitter disappointment for parents to find their children confused, resentful, and withdrawn instead of grateful and delighted by their reunion. The children, too, may be disappointed that their life in Britain is so entirely different from what they had imagined because it is unusual for immigrant children to receive any clear or helpful description of the UK.

Anthea, a seven-year-old West Indian child, and her parents faced many of these problems in an acute form. She came to England when she was six, having lived alone with her grandmother in the West Indies since she was three. Her parents now had a two-year-old son who was placed in a nursery during the day. They both worked extremely long hours and had heavy financial commitments including repaying their fares and a rent of £8 a week for two rooms. These parents, who had looked forward to the arrival of Anthea, were distressed to find her uncommunicative, ignoring, whenever possible, both them and her brother. She appeared uninterested in the expensive clothes her parents had bought for her and her mother was angry when she treated them carelessly. She was particularly anxious that both her children should appear to the neighbours well turned out. Anthea did fairly well at school, but her teachers were sometimes alarmed by her vacant expression and her tendency to stare into space. She was a difficult child to reach and her mother described vividly how she and Anthea would stare at each other in silence.

After school Anthea went to a neighbour until her mother finished work. However, after about three months in England she began to wander off on her way back from school. Her parents would notify the police and then search for Anthea, who would often be found hours later sitting in a park or asleep on a bench. She would not be able to explain why she had wandered nor what she had done. No one could doubt the dreadful anxiety Anthea's parents experienced during these disappearances, and is it not surprising that they felt angry with their daughter for this apparent ingratitude and the embarrassment they felt when police and social workers became concerned with them. The succession of visits to the Child Guidance Clinic, the Care or Protection proceedings, and the supervision of the Children's Department were only partially successful. The grief Anthea felt for her granny and her anger with her parents for apparently deserting her in Jamaica and then replacing her with a son, became clearer.

The anxiety and shame felt by each parent put a strain on their marriage. The wife, dutifully, but resentfully, gave up her job, but Anthea continued to wander. Her parents felt that 'the Government must take her' both as a protection and a punishment. And yet they were ashamed and disappointed at their mysterious failure to be accepted as good parents. Even though the social worker had a very good relationship with Anthea and her parents, even though a workable arrangement was made whereby Anthea was in a small children's home during the week and with her family at week-ends, there remained scars of the wounds which were, for this family, the inevitable result of migration.

Children who are reunited with their parents in their adolescence may also face serious problems of adjustment. As has been described in a previous section, many will be at an educational disadvantage and so may find it hard to obtain satisfactory employment. They are likely to be confused by the way of life of young people in Britain and, perhaps, wish to copy them. This will probably be fiercely resisted by their parents who may well have a poor opinion of the use they see English children making of their independence and the lack of control their parents seem to have over them. They may also rightly fear that their children who are newly arrived in the UK will not understand the constraints on behaviour that do exist and are recognized by children who have lived all their lives in Britain. Advantage may easily be taken of children suffering from this kind of confusion.

Carol Ann, a fifteen-year-old from Guyana, was in such a situation. She was sent for by her mother, partly, it was suspected, because she had become too much of a handful for her grandmother. She was half excited, half frightened by what she found here. Her mother, who had been unmarried when Carol Ann was born, was terrified lest she should 'misbehave'. She demanded all Carol's wages in return for keep and ordered her to be in by six o'clock every night. At first Carol submitted to this. She was, after all, completely ignorant about the ways of this new country. In mid-winter she still wore a long cotton skirt, a thin blouse and a bandanna round her head and her English was hard to understand. The only work which could be found for her was boring and repetitious, the ideal background for her active adolescent fantasy life. She dreamt of becoming another pop-singing Millie. She found a boy-friend who gave her English clothes. She stayed out late (in her mother's opinion); she did not take her boy-friend home; she refused to give her mother all her wages. All this would seem fairly normal to English parents, but Carol's mother was both furious and scared. It is true that her attitude towards her daughter was somewhat Victorian, but it was also true that she had reason to fear for Carol's safety. If she had been in Guyana, Carol would have accepted that she could only have very limited contact with boys and that to do otherwise would seriously compromise her. It is not altogether surprising that her mother screamed 'You will turn her into a prostitute', when a probation officer tried to persuade her to adopt a more liberal attitude. Carol remained resentful of her mother's attempted control, confused by the freedom she envied and wondering what was expected of her by her boy-friend. It is unlikely that it would be easy for her to find someone with whom she could happily settle down. It is also likely that she would be extremely unsure about how to bring up her children in an almost foreign country.

2 *The second generation: younger children* Although those children who have been born in Britain will not have to face the difficulties of separation and reunion, they and their parents face other problems. Some of these are practical. Many immigrant women have to work to make an essential contribution to the family budget. Some, particularly West Indians, may be single and, therefore, the sole wage earners. Like all other working mothers, they have acute difficulties in finding adequate care for their children, some of whom may be looked after in very unsatisfactory conditions, possibly by several different people. Commonwealth students also face problems in the care of their children. Ellis (1971), in an interesting article, has described the attitudes of West African parents in Britain towards the fostering of their young children. For practical reasons, fostering is a necessity, especially since the pursuit of education in the UK involves considerable expense for individuals and families; but also West African parents may see fostering as a positive experience for their children. It is a widespread practice in West African society and can be viewed as a necessary part of a child's education. Furthermore, their belief in the importance of strict discipline of children makes it possible for some West Africans to see any hardship experienced by their offspring as necessary for their training and good for their character. 'A West African may find the kind of psychological insights that are everyday currency to the educated person in Britain irrelevant or very hard to accept. Long, intense, continuous relationships are not so likely to be a normal part of his family ex-

THE STRAINS OF MIGRATION

periences; discontinuities probably are' (Ellis, 1971, p. 23).
Even those parents who realize that fostering in an inadequate environment may hamper the development of
their children may see little practical alternative to this
continued substitute care.

Some parents, however, may be unwilling to take the
risk of placing their children with inadequate daily minders and so choose to work during the hours their husbands or other relatives can be at home. This frequently
involves working early-morning, or late-night, shifts. It is
not unknown for some women to work nearly the whole
night and attempt to care for their families during the
day. They are, of course, exhausted and so unable to give
their young children the stimulation and care they need.
The fathers, on their return from work, are also tired and
unwilling to spend a lot of time with their children who
may, if they are toddlers living in cramped conditions,
spend long hours in their cots with few playthings, since
some immigrant parents see toys as unnecessary luxuries
and not essential to a child's development. Not surprisingly,
children living in these surroundings, with exhausted and
busy parents, will develop more slowly than those with a
more stimulating environment, particularly if their parents
are on their own and, therefore, homesick and depressed.
They may be withdrawn, or apathetic, or unused to making relationships, and their parents may well be disappointed and mystified by their lack of progress.

Prince (1967) has described some acute instances of these
difficulties when young West Indian children have been
referred for medical assessment because it was thought
that their lack of response to various stimuli indicated
deafness, subnormality, or even autism, although many of
the parents felt that the problem was really one of not
wishing to respond rather than inability to do so. Prince
believes that the retardation of such children may be
associated with a gross lack of intellectual, emotional,
and social stimulation, which their parents, particularly

the mothers, who suffer from the exhaustion and depression which are frequently connected with serious social difficulties, are unable to provide.

Social workers have something to contribute to the diagnosis of these problems and in doing so they will be able to lessen parents' fears that their children are physically damaged and, perhaps, help them to tolerate better the children's lack of response. They also need to explain to parents a child's need for stimulation and discuss ways in which it could be provided. Some recently arrived parents may be unaware of neighbouring parks or playgrounds and in their tiredness and loneliness feel unable to venture outside their homes. They may have to be encouraged to go out, perhaps initially in the company of a social worker or voluntary helper, who may also be able to talk with them about play material for their children.

It may be thought that such things are too simple or obvious or even disparaging to the parents concerned, but it is important to remember that only in the last decade or so has there been much public concern about the activities of pre-school children. It is unreasonable to expect parents who have recently arrived from less advanced and child-centred societies to be fully aware of the importance now placed on young children's intellectual and emotional development.

However, a social worker's task is not just educational. In some cases, urgent arrangements should be made for children to attend playgroups, and if their mothers are too confused or exhausted to take much part in them, there should be some flexibility in the pressure put on them to do this. Priorities need to be balanced to allow for the children's urgent need for play and stimulation and for the mothers' need both to see some response in their children and, no less important, to have a short break from them, even though this may, at first sight, appear to contradict the goal of many playgroups, which is to help parents and children to play together and enjoy each other's company.

3 *The second generation: older children* Some of the most complex problems facing immigrant families with older children cluster around the degree of independence these children want and are allowed. This demand to be free of some of the bonds of the family can be a source of anger and concern for their parents because it may be seen as a threat to the structure of the family and a desertion of traditions, which not only are important in themselves but also provide immigrants with security in an unfamiliar country and a link with their native lands. Questions about the extent of older children's independence involve, therefore, a consideration of a family's basic values and beliefs and their view of their future in the country of immigration.

Some parents, particularly mothers, who are lonely and isolated, are also reluctant to allow their children a reasonable measure of independence as they grow up, because they fear that in doing so they will lose them and all that has given some meaning and purpose to their very confined lives in an alien country. Some mothers, too, who have had to leave their other children in their native countries, may in their guilt and sense of loss cling tenaciously to the children still living with them. The children will resent this clinging behaviour but feel guilty if, by trying to withdraw, they add to their mothers' unhappiness. Such parents and children will need a great deal of patient support and understanding from their families and social workers if they are to be able to allow their children some degree of freedom.

Possibly immigrant parents' greatest cause for concern revolves around the discipline of their children and the standards of behaviour they wish them to adopt. Many parents are unimpressed by the independence of older English children and the apparently *laissez-faire* attitudes of their parents. Such methods of child-rearing are totally alien to them and are seen as the origin of much potential unhappiness in their families. And yet they realize that their traditional methods of upbringing are not entirely appropriate for children whose friends and school companions enjoy a much greater degree of independence. Some parents see that some adaptation must be made, but are uncertain how to do this and, for many of them, there is an absence of acceptable models. Most of their compatriots will probably be facing similar difficulties and so there is little common tried experience on which to build. Those who live in the most deprived urban areas may believe that the near delinquent behaviour of many of their neighbours' children is a necessary consequence of more liberal parental attitudes. They may be well aware that their children are being presented with three different models of behaviour—that of their family, their school, and their peers—and are themselves quite at a loss to know whether an acceptable synthesis is possible. Privately, they may envy their children's easier contact with English people and feel humiliated when they act as interpreters for their parents.

(a) Problems of identity and tradition. Many parents' anxieties about their children's behaviour are increased if they feel that they are 'on trial' in an alien country and will be accepted only if they seem to be more than usually successful. Unruly behaviour from their children, therefore, becomes a cause of great concern and anger, particularly if it attracts the attention of public officials whose approval may be seen as important. Added to this anxiety are feelings of sadness and bewilderment when the children are hostile or apathetic about the maintenance of religious and cultural traditions which are an essential part of their parents' lives. Most of the children of immigrant parents have never seen their parents' native lands and may see their customs as eccentric, old-fashioned, and out of place in Britain, rather than as part of the cultural heritage of millions of people in huge countries.

It can seem, therefore, to many parents, particularly those who have not been very successful in establishing themselves economically, that their world, with its close links with other immigrants, holds few attractions for their children and so can have little power over them. Leissner (1969) reports that fathers in poor migrant communities in the USA are especially vulnerable and are likely to be severely criticized and despised by their children for not having made a greater success of their life. Additionally, since the economic and emotional security of many immigrants can depend on their retaining the approval and support of their compatriots, they may look very unsympathetically on behaviour from their children which seems to offend or go against the traditional ways of life.

None the less, particularly after they have been in Britain for some years, some immigrants, and especially their children, may wish for more than just economic security and want to be recognized by, or accepted as part of, the wider community. They will be aware of a double pull on their interests and loyalties and will be unsure whether this can be reconciled with a way of life acceptable to themselves, their compatriots, and long-established residents of the UK. In many respects they are suspended between two cultures.

We do not yet know how far the different immigrant groups will want or be able to adapt to the society in which they now live, nor the extent to which the maintenance of different cultural traditions will be tolerated by their children and the rest of the population. Immigrants and natives feel threatened by each other and since the change they may both have to face is painful, fearful, and frequently resisted, some conflict seems inevitable.

With this uncertain background, at the very least parents are likely to be ambivalent about their children's wish and ability to have some independence from their families and adapt to a more English way of life. Some, however, especially those who feel unhappy and unsettled in Britain, may cling tenaciously to old customs and be disappointed by their failure to maintain their families in these traditional ways and fearful of the consequences.

(b) Adolescents. Most adolescents in European societies go through a period when they question and, perhaps, rebel against their parents' ideals and norms of behaviour in an attempt to establish their own values and identity. Although this pattern of adolescent rebellion may not be so familiar in less advanced countries, it is likely that children whose parents came from the New Commonwealth will be influenced by the behaviour of their peers. The educational system in Britain also encourages, to some extent, a questioning rather than an accepting attitude, and certainly most school teachers expect that many adolescents will reject, temporarily at least, many of their elders' cherished beliefs. Many of the older children of immigrants may resent the traditional attitude of their parents which sees them, on the one hand, as children who owe obedience to their parents and do not need to be consulted when decisions are made about them, and, on the other, as young adults with extensive responsibilities towards the family. Those adolescents whose parents are themselves uncertain about the relevance of some of their values and customs to their life in Britain, especially if they are disappointed by their achievements, have an almost perfect setting in which to act out their rebellion. They know that the constraints on their behaviour are relatively unusual and they are also likely to be aware that their families may be confused, and perhaps disagree amongst themselves, about the nature and extent of these constraints. Their plea for more rights and fewer duties will, therefore, have the support of people within their families and outside.

The strength of these adolescents' position is in itself a danger. Most parents feel threatened by the behaviour and demands of their adolescent children, but immigrant parents are, for all the reasons already described, in a particularly vulnerable position. To what they see as the extreme and even intolerable behaviour of their children, an unwelcome and unnecessary assertion of individuality, they may make a response which is, in its turn, seen by many as unreasonable or excessively strict. In an atmosphere of fear, threat, and mutual recrimination, there is little chance of calm discussion of family problems, and some parents may resort to a method of discipline which, while not so uncommon in their native countries, meets with disapproval in Britain. Threats of physical reprisals or the actual beating of children or locking them up, while not common amongst immigrant families, are sometimes used when they feel in a desperate position; at such moments they are much more fearful than most parents about the consequences of their children's rebellion and can see no alternative way of exercising control over them.

Immigrants are not the only people who panic in this way. The teachers and social workers who are in touch with their children are frequently worried and indignant about the control to which they are subject. They see children born and educated in Britain as needing, and rightly expecting, a way of life similar to that of their peers and so they often identify strongly with the child under their supervision. Understandable though this identification may be, it is not necessarily helpful to either the child or his parents because it ignores the complexities and tensions which are an inevitable part of the relationship between immigrant parents and their children. The heat and anger engendered in disagreements and the extreme positions adopted by the persons involved may seem unusual, but they are intimately connected with the severe demands that migration makes on a family.

There is no reason to suppose that the majority of families, where relationships are affectionate and well established, will not ride out the storm of conflict between the generations, painful and threatening though this will be, in the same way that they overcome the other serious problems of adjustment which face all migrants. Those families that do not manage to do this may be subject to additional serious tensions and problems, some of which may have existed before the family's migration. What social workers and teachers must realize is that the family group provides immigrants, more so than most people, with a basic source of security which cannot easily be replaced. Those who have had close contact with immigrant families of many nationalities have noticed that children often accept the differences in their lives in and outside the family and make good adjustment to the dual demands on them, even though this may only be achieved after some pain and conflict. It is therefore important to consider what alternative way of life faces the child of immigrant parents who makes a break with his family and whether such a child has the resources to survive and flourish away from it. Although some children may need to make such a break and be able to establish themselves more independently, it is likely that they will be exceptional. The following case study illustrates many aspects of this conflict between the generations.

Parents and children in conflict: a case study

The Williamsons, a West Indian family from St Kitts, became known to the Probation Service when James, aged fifteen, appeared in a Juvenile Court charged with taking and driving away a car together with some other coloured boys. Mr Williamson, his stepfather, had been very angry and upset in court and said that he wanted James to be sent away, together with Beverley, his sister aged sixteen. He gave a furious and somewhat incoherent account of her insolence and rudeness, her refusal to give her parents her earnings, her obstinacy about making dates with boys her parents did not know, and the late hours she kept.

Before visiting the family during the remand for social enquiry reports, the Probation Office was telephoned by the Health Visitor who knew Mrs Williamson well. She described her as very depressed since the birth of her youngest child, now only a few months old, partly because she was no longer able to go out to work and so get some relief from the tensions in the family which had been developing for some time. The Health Visitor said that she had been concerned about Beverley and James but had not approached the Children's Department as Mr and Mrs Williamson had been very against this. The Health Visitor also told the Probation Officer that although Beverley and James were Mrs Williamson's illegitimate children, their stepfather, Mr Williamson, had taken full responsibility for them, but there were times when he threatened to disown them. James was said to have had some severe beatings from Mr Williamson; and Beverley, to have on occasions been locked in the house. The Health Visitor described Mr Williamson as rather puritanical and rigid in his attitudes and stricter than Mrs Williamson. There had been some stormy disagreements between them about the control of the children, and Mrs Williamson was apparently afraid that if she asserted herself too much, Mr Williamson would carry out his threats to desert the whole family.

Like the Child Care Officer who visited the Khan family, the Probation Officer's first meeting with the Williamsons was difficult. He felt that Mr Williamson's accounts of Beverley's and James's misdeeds were exaggerated and he was somewhat put off by his constant referral to Biblical texts to support his point of view. The family Bible occupied a central position in the living room, and the Probation Officer learnt that Mr Williamson was an active member of the local Pentecostal Church, whose congregation was composed largely of West Indians. Although Mrs Williamson was less vociferous in her complaints about James and Beverley, she described graphically the trials she and her husband experienced in bringing them to Britain when they were six and seven and in establishing the family. Undoubtedly, they had been very successful in this respect; they had a comfortably furnished flat and Mr Williamson had recently been promoted to the position of foreman carpenter; Mrs Williamson had been a senior ward maid. Both felt that their children's behaviour would cast a very bad light on them, that they would be shamed in front of their church friends, and that their employers would be disgusted if they learnt of James's court appearance.

Throughout this discussion, Mr and Mrs Williamson showed themselves to be very ambivalent about their view of the English way of life, describing their children's acquaintances as thieves and prostitutes, their parents as lazy, and the schools as a breeding ground of the difficulties they were now experiencing with James and Beverley. They much preferred the customs of St Kitts, where children respected their parents and showed responsibility for their family. At the same time, they spoke with pride of their achievements and of the good progress at school of their next two children; they thought it likely that they would get some higher education and hoped that their daughter would be a nurse and their son a television engineer. Mr Williamson also showed that he was very aware of, and indignant about, discrimination against coloured people, implying at times that they must stand together and fight for their rights. None the less, he was anxious about James's association with the coloured boys with whom he was charged, as he thought they were under the influence of a student who was apparently trying to get together a group of young coloured people to draw attention to the predicament of immigrants and fight for their rights. Mr Williamson thought that his motives and methods were dubious and would reflect badly on coloured people. He was adamant thoughout the discussion that he would no longer be responsible for Beverley and James and that the 'government would have to take them away, school them, and punish them!' He refused to discuss any other alternative.

When the Probation Officer met Beverley and James, he found them sullen, resentful, and angry with their parents, particularly their stepfather. He thought that their complaints about his very strict control were quite reasonable, realizing that they were expected to behave in a quite different way to their white peers. He was particularly worried about James's account of the beatings his father had given him, and privately had grave doubts about the possibility of their remaining at home with their parents. He probably conveyed this doubt to Beverley and James, who said they wanted to leave home, although they did not know where or how they could live on their own.

Later during the remand, the Probation Officer was told by the police that they had taken Beverley home very late at night after she had been found wandering around the streets. She had apparently climbed out of the window of the room in which Mr Williamson had locked her after a family row. The Probation Officer was very worried and wondered whether he should recommend a Care Order for James and ask the Children's Department to find a hostel place for Beverley. However, on balance he thought it preferable to try a period of supervision, and James was placed on probation; it was agreed that Beverley should see the Probation Officer on a voluntary basis. Although Mrs Williamson seemed quite relieved by this decision, Mr Williamson was not happy about it and during the first few months the Probation Officer sometimes despaired of any modification in his attitudes. Beverley and James continued to be pretty rebellious, in the opinion of their parents, and the Probation Officer, too, thought there was some deterioration in their behaviour. After one particularly bad row, he arranged for Beverley to stay at a voluntary hostel. This did not work out as well as expected, and although she now had a great deal more independence, she seemed listless and lonely, returning home frequently.

The Probation Officer maintained close contact with Mr

and Mrs Williamson, seeing them both together and separately. Slowly quite a close and warm relationship developed in which the Williamsons discussed their life in St Kitts, their disappointments at the problems they found awaiting them in Britain, as well as their anxiety about their children. They were grateful for the efforts made by the Probation Officer to get James into good employment and agreed to allow both him and Beverley to be introduced to a Church Youth Club. With the assistance of the Health Visitor, the Probation Officer also helped Mrs Williamson to return to part-time work, leaving her baby in the care of a good daily minder. While recognizing that this was not an ideal situation, he realized that Mrs Williamson greatly needed the outlet work could give her and with this would become less anxious and depressed about her relationship with her husband and children. In the course of her discussions with the Probation Officer, Mrs Williamson described her sorrow at having to leave Beverley and James in St Kitts at the time when she came to Britain. She also said that she had not realized, or wanted to face, the extent of their confusion and unhappiness after their parting from their aunt and uncle and their reunion with their parents. She emphasized that she did not want Beverley 'to follow her ways' by having illegitimate children. She recognized that this was much disapproved of in England and that the care of such children would be extremely difficult. Both Mr and Mrs Williamson seemed aware that their children's future in Britain would be uncertain and fraught with difficulties; nevertheless, laying great stress on the support the members of the family could give each other, and the strength and self-respect they would all derive from strict adherence to their interpretation of a Christian code of behaviour, they seemed confident that Beverley and James would be able to cope. In this more relaxed, good-humoured atmosphere, the Probation Officer came to understand the strengths of their outlook, although he was not always in sympathy with it, and thought it unlikely that Beverley and James, or indeed the other children, would want to abide by all the high standards their parents set for them.

As Mr and Mrs Williamson came to trust the Probation Officer more, the tension between them and Beverley and James eased. Although both the older children continued at times to complain of the constraints on their behaviour, they also seemed absorbed in activities outside their home, both at work and at their Youth Club. Beverley returned to live at home. The Probation Officer realized that his original pessimistic view of the relationship between the parents and the children had not fully taken into account the strengths in the family and the support and protection it provided. He also thought that his initial extreme sympathy for Beverley's and James's predicament, which arose partly from comparing it with that of white children, had not been particularly helpful.

The Probation Officer, Beverley, and James together gained a good deal from taking part in a discussion group arranged by a youth leader especially for young people who felt they were having difficulties with their parents. At times this group consisted almost entirely of coloured adolescents who seemed to get some help from sharing and comparing their resentments about the degree of their parents' control. Given this relief, they were also able to talk perceptively about their parents' difficulties and uncertainties, and showed some acceptance that their pattern of family life would differ in some ways from that of many white people. There were, of course, some young people unable or unwilling to recognize and appreciate their parents' situation, and they were extremely envious of the degree of freedom allowed to white children in the group. The group leader was worried lest this envy should contribute to a deterioration in the behaviour of these coloured youths. On the whole, however, this sharing of experiences seemed helpful to everyone, with some white children being able to recognize that their parents were relatively liberal, and the moderate coloured children upbraiding their more extreme companions for demands which they thought unreasonable in view of their parents' predicament. Although there was some antagonism between the coloured and white young people, there were also periods of mutual sharing and understanding arising from a recognition of common problems. Both the youth leader and the Probation Officer made contact with the parents of the children in the group in an effort to prevent them from feeling isolated or threatened by their children's meetings. They hoped eventually to form a similar parents' discussion group.

Eventually, the Probation Officer began to act as negotiator for the Williamson family, and rules concerning Beverley's and James's activities were discussed with them and their parents and compromises reached which allowed for some modification of the demands of both sides. It was only possible for the Probation Officer to do this because of the trust all the Williamsons placed in him, although it must be admitted that he sometimes found the dual pull on him exhausting. He was also uncertain about the extent to which he should exert his authority, of which the family had an exaggerated view, implying at times that they thought they must abide by his views as though they were the orders of 'the government'. Although the family continued to have some quite fierce rows no one, including the Probation Officer, took the threats and abuse that were hurled around so seriously that they resorted to panic activity. There seemed some confidence that these rows would blow over and that reasonable relationships would be re-established. The Probation Officer thought this pattern might continue with the younger children, although possibly in a less extreme form as the family grew more sure of its ability to survive serious tensions amongst its members.

It is possible that this relatively happy outcome could not have been achieved if, in their early childhood, Beverley and James had been separated from their parents for a longer period and reunited only in adolescence. In other cases, where family conflict is more serious and chronic, both parents and children may need to be apart from each other for a period. However, it remains important for social workers faced with this situation to keep a close contact with the child away from home and his parents, however unlikely seems the possibility of successful reunion. In spite of violent threats of everlasting separation, the very isolation and loneliness of many coloured people may mean that eventually they will want and need the support and companionship of their relatives.

Migrants' choice and governments' responsibility

What sort of place could this England be that everyone who went there came back a rich man and lived in such luxurious ease? I began to realise that there might be places in the world free of the drudgery and poverty which I saw around me...

If someone had told me 'Rampal, some day you will indeed go to England and you will suffer much unhappiness there' I would not have believed it ... my mind was filled only with optimistic thoughts for my future...

Most of the Indians who came here are like me, village people in need of work, and they come here to earn money, not just for the fun of the trip. If anyone says he's here for a holiday, he is telling a lie. Would anyone work in another's house if he had plenty to eat in his own? Why else should we leave the country where we were born and where we have our land and kin? (Sharma, 1971, pp. 55, 73, 109).

Given all the personal and social difficulties with which migrants must contend, it is not surprising that some people wonder why so many are prepared to undertake such a risky enterprise. This question is sometimes asked as a preliminary to suggestions that immigrants should return to their native countries if they do not like their new found circumstances. Since so few seem prepared to do this, it is assumed, often correctly, that however difficult their lot, their life after migration must in many respects be preferable to their experiences in their native countries. Why, then, should the countries of immigration be concerned to protect the interests of their new citizens? It is also suggested that potential migrants might be deterred from leaving their native countries if they could be fully informed of the hardships that await them.

These are important questions asked by most people who are concerned with immigrants, but only rarely are they rationally debated. This is primarily because in public discussion they frequently form part of the armoury of reactionary groups and are used to stir up feeling against immigrants. And yet these questions have to be considered calmly if individuals and organizations are to devise policies which are strong and effective because they represent their firm conviction.

In the first place, as the previous chapters have indicated, migration must be seen in the context of gross differences in the wealth of nations. For centuries some countries have been the receivers and others the sources of migrant labour. As governments are drawn closer together by political and industrial treaties and as communications improve, no advanced country can expect to be immune from immigration and many will encourage it. In some less advanced countries, as the next chapter will show, there is a long tradition of the more enterprising families seeking to improve their circumstances by migration, and undoubtedly many of them achieve their ambitions. Against this background, an immigrant family must be understood not as courageously, if perversely, deciding to inflict misery on itself in the pursuit of economic gain but rather as being caught up in world-wide economic and political developments. Disillusioned though many people are with the viability of the nuclear family in Western society, we do not blame those families that follow this pattern; nor are we surprised that the majority have not weighed its losses and gains. Life in an advanced industrial economy leaves most of them with no choice. Many families, if they are to survive and prosper, have equally little choice about their migration. This in itself may place an almost intolerable strain on them.

For such people, return to their native countries will usually be economically impossible not only for themselves but for their relatives who have sponsored their migration and are dependent on money sent back home. It will also be socially impossible, for to return in poverty would be to admit failure. There are many pressures on migrants to paint a cheerful picture of their circumstances. Furthermore, in the early days of their settlement, in their isolation from the wider society, they may not be fully aware of the extent of their deprivation or the poor chance there is to escape from it. It is their children who will be more conscious of being trapped in a vicious circle. It is also difficult for immigrants to convey to their relatives back home the changes in family relationships which are some of the most painful consequences of migration. Often these can only be understood with hindsight and to admit to them may bring shame and recrimination on a family.

In these circumstances, efforts to inform people of the risks of migration—while they might succeed in reducing the aspirations of many immigrants and, therefore, the shock they experience on their arrival in a new country— will probably not deter them. Not only are family pressures and expectations too strong for this, but the effectiveness of information programmes will also be countered by the obvious differences in the wealth and opportunity of the advanced and backward nations.

Given that many peoples' circumstances do improve after their migration, even though the price of this improvement is great, the answer to the question about the responsibility of the receiving country for its new citizens is based on expediency and morality. Industrial nations cannot afford to have in their cities permanently deprived minorities. At best, this is a waste of valuable human resources; at worst, it can result in grave tensions which may find their release through violence. We also have to acknowledge that while immigrants may expect exploitation, this cannot, in justice, be their children's inheritance. Nor can we condone suffering, and allow it to continue with the excuse that immigrants were not forced to leave their native countries and, comparatively speaking, have improved their lot by doing so. What return are advanced industrial countries prepared to make from the labour of migrants, who, explicitly or implicitly, have been invited to contribute to their economy? Our beliefs about equality face their most stringent test in the views we adopt about the needs and rights of immigrants and their families.

Colour and migration

'Out of the blackest part of my soul, across the zebra striping of my mind, surges this desire to be suddenly white' (Fanon, 1970, p. 46).

Previous sections have shown the special problems coloured people face in Britain as in many other predominantly white countries. Immigrants and their children soon become aware of the common association of colour with poverty, lack of ability, and general deprivation. To some people, it seems as though their colour, rather than anything else, condemns them to the status of second- and third-class citizens and is the chief or only barrier to their obtaining a more satisfactory position in society. Many coloured people, particularly West Indians, set a high store on light skin colour and see this, often quite realistically, as a passport to better jobs and a higher status.

From an early age, the children of immigrants from the New Commonwealth are likely to be aware of their colour and its negative associations. Goodman (1964) is only one of many researchers who have found that even children as young as three and four, particularly if they are Negro, have a clear perception of colour and social attribute and are aware of patterns of racial discrimination. It is probable, therefore, that even in their primary schools coloured children may come to perceive, however dimly, that some people think that they are inferior. As they grow older, and particularly as they look for employment and companionship with the opposite sex, resentment and hostility between whites and coloured young people increase. Some coloured young people, aware of this potential conflict, try hard to avoid confrontations with white people. As Hall (1967, pp. 9-10) describes it: 'through the hostile [twilight] areas, coloured youngsters walk in groups and avoid trouble. Our cities are full of young coloured citizens of Britain trying to tiptoe through society.'

In their anger and distress, some young people try to reject their colour or racial characteristics. It has been observed that when coloured and white children are brought up together, coloured children sometimes try to make themselves a lighter colour by excessive washing or scraping their skins. Some seem to believe that, as cygnets change into swans, so as they get older they will turn white. Some older Negro girls try to straighten their hair and bleach their skin to a lighter colour. More seriously, they may reject their parents, whom they see as having made them coloured, together with any customs they regard as associated with coloured people and, therefore, inferior and the reason for their failure in an increasingly competitive and segregated world. They wish only to be seen as totally English and may indulge in fantasies about their parentage, believing that a number of their ancestors were white. They may despise friendship with coloured young people and yearn for friendships with white boys and girls, although it is quite likely that they will be rejected by them. At a very vulnerable stage of development these young people will have few people with whom to identify, and their parents, often deeply hurt by their children's rejection and accusations, may not be able to help them.

Some coloured young people have found security in organizations associated with Black Power ideals. The value such organizations place on colour and the culture of countries, particularly Africa, from which the ancestors of many immigrants originated, is important in helping young coloured people not to despise themselves and their background. Some, too, will be encouraged by the ideology which calls for more power for coloured people, as this provides a welcome alternative to an existence in which coloured people seem always to take second place to whites.

Because some Black Power organizations have been associated with extremism, many people have feared them and regretted their development in Britain. They ignore the fact that the values of Black Power may be extremely important for a group of demoralized young people who see little future for themselves and few channels for their resentment. The adoption of such values does not inevitably mean taking up positions of extreme hostility to white people or believing that amibitions can only be achieved by violence and the assumption of all the means of power by coloured people. These attitudes develop only when an underprivileged group meets apathy or intransigent resistance to its demands for a more equitable society. None the less, those immigrant parents who wish to establish their families as peacefully and as easily as possible in the UK find it hard to sympathize with their children's association with Black Power organizations. Equally, they are often painfully aware of the handicap of their colour and at a loss to know how to influence their children's attitudes towards the society in which they live.

In a study of black families in the USA, Billingsley (1968), writes perceptively of the dilemma facing many Negro parents. He points out that it is quite mistaken to see colour and deprivation as necessarily associated, since many coloured families are successfully established and have a resilience and adaptability which have helped them to survive in a nation hostile to them. None the less, these families are aware that for generations they have been treated as inferior and that their children, even more than they, will resent this and protest against it. Are they to be encouraged to do this? In a violent society such aggressive self-assertion can cost people their liberty and their lives. Even in a more peaceful environment, those who protest loudly can be identified as troublemakers, not to be trusted with responsibility. Those who are ambitious to establish themselves successfully in a society unwilling to accommodate itself to minority groups take risks if they also choose to protest against its inequalities. Understandably, some immigrant families wonder whether these risks are justified. And yet, the alternative to protest is also dangerous, because it involves people accepting inferior status, thrust on them as right and justified. Ultimately, this means self-contempt and apathy. Young coloured people are faced, therefore, with a situation in which both acquiescence to injustice and resistance to it involves risks of self-destruction. Their parents have to grapple with the problem of building up their children's confidence and assuring them of their worth without inspiring in them hatred for the society which discriminates against them. Those who can solve this dilemma frequently possess remarkable self-control and draw strength from religious or philosophical convictions.

Some older immigrants may have come to accept the inequalities in the treatment of different racial groups, as in their view, an easier and immediately more profitable course than protest against this injustice. However, their children, possibly because of better education or greater confidence, will be unwilling to tolerate any differences in the treatment of coloured and white people. Their demand for equal rights and opportunities, together with a changing political climate which allows for conflict rather than cohesion in society, is likely in the next few years to heighten the tension felt by young coloured people between their wish to protest and the pressures on them to acquiesce.

Social workers must be aware that it is this conflict which will contribute in no small way to the tension in immigrant families and the turbulence experienced by many individuals. They will not be able to prevent or remove it, but it may be their job to help families to clarify some of the issues which underlie their anxiety, anger, and confusion. It will also be important for social workers, who are familiar with the dilemmas facing coloured families, to make these known to their colleagues and others who do not understand them and resent and fear what they consider to be the unreasonable behaviour of some coloured people. The outcome of the tensions experienced by many immigrant families is not yet known, but it is clear that social workers will need special training, and must accustom themselves to working in situations which sometimes involve fierce conflict and great pain, and where easy and cohesive solutions cannot be expected.

Future developments amongst young coloured people

There are many families in Britain, whose ancestors came originally from Ireland or Europe, who regard themselves, and are seen by others, as British in every way. They are widely distributed throughout the different strata of society. However, only a few coloured families have lived in Britain for more than fifty years, and it is not easy to generalize from their experiences in attempts to predict the pattern of life of the children and grandchildren of migrant families. None the less, the evidence so far is not encouraging, particularly if coloured people continue to be concentrated in the poorest urban areas. Recent studies of parts of Cardiff and Liverpool in which coloured people have lived for many years and suffered great hardship, suggest that young coloured people feel uneasy and rejected in a predominantly white society. Denied many of the opportunities open to white people, especially those in more prosperous areas, many lack ambition and do not realize their potential. They justify their eagerness to leave school by pointing out that they will anyway have little chance of good employment. Although these young people have some social contact with their white peers, they feel insecure and expect to meet greater prejudice if they move far outside their home areas. They regret being cut off from the main stream of city life, but see it as an inevitable consequence of being coloured in a white city. Especially when their parents regard themselves as British, these young people feel they have neither a place in their native society nor an alternative culture with which to identify.

In a particularly difficult position are the children of mixed white and coloured parentage. They frequently seem to be rejected, belonging to no identifiable group. This is probably one reason why the children of mixed unions are over-represented in children's homes. Those who remain with their families can also face serious difficulties. Writing more than twenty years ago, Little (1947) found that some children with a white mother and coloured father faced a conflict of loyalties and that to avoid this, many of them tended to withdraw and avoid identification with either parent. He thinks that this contributed to an attitude of detachment in which emotional and intellectual problems were avoided and to shiftless, sometimes negative, behaviour. It is likely that these young people will feel more than any others that they live in neither an alien nor a local culture and, although they may well have adopted the prevailing values of the area, they will realize that they probably have little chance of abiding by them.

Some young people whose parents are both coloured may also try to adopt this attitude of detachment from their families and from the world outside in an attempt to avoid painful conflicts. This will be unhelpful if it prevents them from taking the risks involved in commitment to important long-term relationships, thus missing the satisfaction and security these provide, and being handicapped in grappling with the pressures and competition of an urban society. Social workers will probably find it difficult to establish helpful relationships with people caught in this dilemma, but they need to attempt this as, in doing so, they may be able to help young coloured people explore the reasons for their resistance to attachment and dependence and offer them the opportunity of a bridging relationship between themselves, their parents, and other important people in their environment.

Some possible reactions

The predicament of the descendants of coloured immigrants in Britain could result in two possible reactions, apathy or alienation from, and hostility towards, the society in which they live. Describing a retreatist response, Merton (1968, p. 244) quotes from an earlier study:

> One prominent type of apathy is the loss of involvement in a previously sought cultural goal, such as occurs when continued striving results in persistent and seemingly unavoidable frustration. The loss of central life goals leaves the individual in a social vacuum, without focal direction or meaning. But another crucial kind of apathy seems to emerge from conditions of great normative complexity and/or rapid social change, when individuals are pushed this way and that by numerous conflicting norms and goals, until the person is literally disorientated and demoralised, unable to secure a firm commitment to a set of norms that he can feel as self-consistent.

Although this would seem to describe the position of some of the descendants of coloured immigrants, it is likely to be counteracted by their ambitions, their sense of justice, and, to some extent, their education. They are aware that the inequalities they face are deeply regretted by many people and that some attempts have been made through the law and social policy to redress these with varying degrees of success. Some will, therefore, be encouraged to fight for their rights possibly by attacking those whom they see as standing in their way or, alternatively, by using established channels of protest to draw attention to their predicament and secure social justice. A number of factors will determine the course taken by individual immigrants, but the influence of social workers who, together with teachers, may be the only representatives of established authority with whom coloured people have any degree of intimate contact, could be an important factor in determining the choice made. Their attitudes, and the work they are able to do in helping coloured families and influencing those people who have power to improve their circumstances more substantially, will be an indication of the extent to which immigrants and their families may hope realistically for some solution to their difficulties within the existing political and social structure.

The dilemma for the social worker is similar to the one facing many immigrant parents. He will be aware of the paralysing effects of apathy and may wish to help coloured people to assert themselves and claim their rights; but he may also fear that such encouragement will unleash angry and hostile behaviour from coloured people which may ultimately rebound on them. He must remember that however distressed he is by the inequalities he sees, and however much he may influence his clients, the final decision about protest or acceptance must rest with them; and there will be some people who believe that the price of protest, or even of claiming their rights, for example under the Race Relations Act, is too great. The social worker must tread a delicate path between helping people to identify and protest against what they regard as intolerable and encouraging them to modify some of their attitudes and behaviour in an attempt to improve their position in society.

All these vicissitudes, which are the expected lot of many migrant families and their descendants, usually become overwhelmingly only when they are accompanied by the burden of multiple deprivation described in the previous chapter. The situation in many American cities provides us with the most horrifying evidence of the results of the neglect of poverty and discrimination and the inevitable isolation and deterioration of the Negro family. Although there are important differences between American and British experience, we should not believe that we are immune from the appalling problems Brown (1969, p. 8) describes in his vivid but sickening account of his childhood and youth in Harlem. He was well aware of the hopelessness experienced by many people for whom migration to the city had once held the promise of a better life.

It seems that Cousin Willie, in his lying haste, had neglected to tell the folks down home about one of the most important aspects of the promised land: it was a slum ghetto. There was a tremendous difference in the way life was lived up North. There were too many people full of hate and bitterness crowded into a dirty, stinky, uncared for closet-size section of a great city ... The children of these disillusioned coloured pioneers inherited the total lot of their parents—the disappointments, the anger. To add to their misery, they had little hope of deliverance. For where does one run to when he's already in the promised land?

5

The social and cultural background of immigrants

The recognition in recent years of the great differences between the various groups of coloured immigrants in Britain and the extent to which many of them wish to retain their cultural identity, has led to an increasing interest on the part of English people in their customs and social background. Most social workers now realize that this knowledge will greatly influence their understanding and treatment of the problems of their immigrant clients.

There are, however, some risks in focusing too exclusively on the pattern of life in the immigrants' native countries. In the first place, such an approach assumes that culture is static, and fails to take account of the adaptation which many people make, willingly or unwillingly, in the course of their migration. We do not yet know the extent of this adaptation, which will depend partly on the immigrants' expectation of permanent or temporary settlement and partly on the areas in which they live and the nature of their contact with native people. The previous chapter has shown how immigrant families are already facing, and partly accepting, some significant changes in the pattern of their family relationships and in their attitudes which would be unfamiliar or shocking to many of their compatriots who have not emigrated. Under pressure from the old world and the new, they both share and are influenced by a migrant culture of adaptation. About this culture, which will vary from group to group, so far we know little.

Second, in the absence of particular information about the background of those individuals who do decide to emigrate, we do not know how far they can be seen as typical of those living in similar social and economic circumstances. Unlike the early migration from Ireland, when nearly every family could expect to have at least one member overseas, only a small minority of people from the West Indies, India, and Pakistan emigrate. Although a tradition of migration seems to have been established amongst some groups of people for several generations, we do not know exactly what influences a particular family or village to undertake this enterprise nor how they are seen by their fellow countrymen. However, it is probably safe to assume that they represent some of the most ambitious and least satisfied members of their society, and are also unusual in their wish and ability to do something fairly drastic to improve their circumstances.

Third, since the process of migration often involves a transfer from rural to urban society before an individual leaves his native country, an immigrant who came originally from a peasant community may have some experience of urban life before he comes to Britain. His way of life and attitudes cannot, therefore, be understood solely in terms of the values and customs of a peasant society. Sharma's (1971) vivid account of the experience of an Indian migrant family illustrates well all these points.

It is therefore unwise, in attempting to understand the way of life of immigrants in Britain, to rely too heavily on accounts of the cultural background of their native countries without taking into account the way in which these customs and beliefs have been interpreted by them. Social workers will need to supplement and expand the basic background information they have by discussing with immigrants their views of the differences and similarities in their style of life before and after their migration. In doing this, the social workers should not be reluctant to admit their ignorance or confusion about certain aspects of immigrants' lives, because not only can it be helpful for some immigrants to reflect on their experiences in an attempt to trace some continuity in their lives; but some also appreciate the opportunity of being in the position of providers rather than receivers of information. Such requests for information can be seen as one attempt on the part of the receiving society to understand and, therefore, make some adaptation to its immigrant members. In gathering these impressions, social workers could obtain some valuable insights into the patterns of life of immigrant communities which have not yet been fully documented, although they must remember that inevitably they are in touch with that small minority of people who are unusual in that they have been unable to solve their own difficulties unaided.

West Indians in Britain

To go into more detail—tell you where he come from originally, whether he six foot tall or five foot six, whether he have big eyes and small nose—what difference it make to you? All you interested in that he black—to English people every black man look the same. And to tell you he came from Trinidad and not Jamaica—them two places a thousand miles apart—won't make any difference to you, because to Englishers the West Indies is the West Indies, and if a man say he come from Tobago or St. Lucia or Grenada, you none the wiser (Selvon, 1965, p. 24).

Partly because West Indians are the oldest established of the coloured immigrant groups, and partly because their common language makes them more approachable to English people, more has been written about their social background and their settlement in Britain. Some West Indian novelists have also written well about the experience of newly arrived immigrants in Britain. However, the rapidly changing circumstances surrounding immigration mean that studies of West Indian settlement, made less than a decade ago, may now be outdated. Nevertheless, enough is now known about West Indian immigrants and their families to make possible a fairly good understanding of their position in British society, the complexities of which make them perhaps the most vulnerable of the immigrant groups. For these reasons, it is both possible and necessary to write at some length about them.

In 1966, West Indians formed the largest single group of Commonwealth immigrants. Although over half of them came from Jamaica, there were emigrants from several other islands. Selvon's somewhat bitter remark highlights the great difficulty that exists in making generalizations about the social background of people whose homelands consist of a large number of islands, of varying sizes, which have been influenced by different foreign powers—English, French, Spanish, and American—and are now at varying stages of economic and political development. Although it will probably be impossible for most English people to have much detailed knowledge about the islands of the West Indies, they should show an awareness that they appreciate that these differences exist and that there is sometimes rivalry between West Indians from different islands, who resent being seen as a single national group with similar background and aspirations.

It is also important to realize that in the West Indies several different patterns of family life can be identified, with variations depending partly on social class and national background. In many of the islands, people whose ancestors came originally from Africa, Europe, and India live in relatively close contact with each other, and although there has been considerable inter-marriage, the styles of life of various groups may follow very different patterns. For example, the family life of a middle-class West Indian of African descent may be identical to that of a white West Indian whose ancestors came originally from Europe. It will, however, be very different from the life familiar to many working-class coloured West Indians, although amongst this group, too, different styles of life can be identified.

There is a considerable literature dealing with the structure of the West Indian family, and sociologists and anthropologists disagree about its complexities. Most of these studies have focused on the working class. Although certain patterns emerge from these studies which seem familiar to those social workers who have West Indian clients, it is unwise to rely too heavily on these accounts not only for the reasons already outlined but also because, as various studies have indicated, a substantial proportion of West Indian immigrants are skilled men who in the West Indies would have seen themselves as belonging to the upper working and lower middle class. However, since many of them have been unable to obtain similar work in Britain, they have taken jobs which place them disproportionately amid the lowest socio-economic groups. West Indians are also some of the worst housed immigrants, and in these respects, particularly in view of their lengthier settlement in the UK, they represent one of the least successful of the coloured immigrant groups. None the less, their identifications and expectations still reflect middle-class values as they understand them. They may, therefore, feel strongly that they do not wish to be associated with the West Indian or English working-class style of life, and may naturally be upset that their immigration has meant a decline in social status.

The influences of slavery and colonization

'I am talking of millions of men who have been skilfully injected with fear, inferiority complexes, trepidation, servility, despair, abasement' (Césaire, 1955, p. 22).

Bearing in mind earlier reservations, there are some patterns of relationship and family life, and some social attitudes, which it is helpful for social workers to understand. Most of these have their origin either in the system of slavery, which was common in the West Indies until the middle of the nineteenth century, or they have developed under the influence of colonial government which, until recently, dominated West Indian affairs. The institutions of slavery have left four important legacies for many working-class West Indians whose ancestors were originally brought from Africa to work on the plantations in the seventeenth and eighteenth centuries.

1 *Illegitimacy and family life* In the first place, the rules forbidding slaves to maintain their tribal customs or adopt a European style of marriage resulted in the absence of most of those institutions regarded as essential to family life and, in particular, in the systematic denial of the role of the Negro man as a husband and father. Although slaves were encouraged to procreate, their children belonged to the slave owners who had only limited obligations towards them, with the major responsibility for their upbringing resting with their mothers; a child's biological father had no rights or duties towards it. Against this background one characteristic pattern of West Indian family life began to emerge in which women were forced to take an independent role and could rely on little regular support from the fathers of their illegitimate children. The West Indian illegitimacy rate has remained high, over 70 per cent in some islands, and so this plight is familiar to many West Indian women, who have to depend heavily on the help of their female relatives to care for their children while they support the family financially. These matriarchal family units may consist of a grandmother and her female children and grandchildren to which a number of men may be attached on a more or less casual basis, but whose rights and duties will be ill defined. The children in these families have, therefore, to rely almost entirely on their female relatives for their upbringing, and Lamming's vivid phrase 'my mother who fathered me' (1953, p. 11) points to the dual

responsibility of their mothers.

2 *Patterns of marriage* This style of life is recognized as far from ideal by most West Indians, but has been greatly influenced and perpetuated by another legacy of slavery, that is the association of a Christian or a European style of marriage with property and social position. In their inferior and degrading position, slaves were well aware of the relationship of mutual rights and obligations that existed between slave owners and other powerful people in the colonies and their wives. Whatever may have been the private infidelity of these husbands towards their wives, they recognized their financial and social obligations towards them and their children. The mistresses of the plantations were influential people, but they acknowledged their dependence on their husbands and the loyalty and obedience due to them. Their relationship provided a model, however distant and unattainable for the slaves, which was associated with freedom and respectability.

This Victorian style of family life was also held up as the ideal in the teachings of the Christian missionaries who were influential amongst the slaves after Emancipation. In the eyes of many Christians, the Negroes represented the noble savage whose way of life would in many respects be uncivilized and who could only rarely, and with great personal effort, attain a style of life which could command the respect of Europeans. Some of these attitudes must have been internalized by the emancipated slaves and their descendants who saw marriage as involving the economic ability of a couple to set up home on their own, for the woman to give up work, and for her husband, now the dominant and responsible partner, to support his family financially, thus at last being in a position to make important decisions and command the respect of his immediate relatives.

Marriage for many poor West Indians is, therefore, a state to be achieved by a couple who may have lived together for a number of years and have several children, and it may represent the culmination of their efforts to establish themselves economically and socially. Not surprisingly, this delay in the West Indies of such a legal and binding union leads very often to a number of preliminary or 'trial' relationships. Sometimes these are very casual affairs which may result in illegitimate children, for whom their fathers feel only spasmodic responsibility; but they can also be faithful cohabitations in which the couple shares responsibility for the children. In these circumstances the woman is expected to contribute financially to the family and, therefore, usually enjoys greater independence than if she were married. In both marriage and cohabitation, each partner is quite likely to have children by another union. When these children live with the couple, some mutual responsibility for them is usually recognized, but, as is shown in the case of the Williamson family, they can be a source of friction and a reminder of a less successful and more insecure past.

3 *Child-rearing practices* The relationships between West Indian children, both legitimate and illegitimate, and their parents and older relatives are reminiscent of those which existed between some Victorian parents and their children. They also reflect the ways in which poor coloured West Indians were treated by those who have exercised authority over them both in a domestic and public context.

West Indians acknowledge their financial responsibility for their children, and either the mothers or fathers are at pains to discharge this. However, in return, they demand their dutiful obedience and respect and often set aside a number of household tasks for them from an early age. Children are not consulted about decisions affecting them or their families because they are seen as 'not understanding', and possibly not even caring, by their parents who, like their Victorian forebears, are not always aware of the extent of children's feelings. Expression of their opinions or assertion of their independence is often described as 'rudeness' and is much frowned upon; especially on social occasions, children, often beautifully dressed in a rather old-fashioned style, are expected to behave like miniature, but mute, adults. Although treated indulgently as babies, as they grow older they are frequently subject to a discipline consisting of orders, threats, and occasional chastisement which can be both harsh and inconsistent. In this way, as with many English working-class children, their ideas of right and wrong may not be internalized or reasoned, but may depend very much on the surrounding circumstances and the presence of people recognized as powerful.

4 *Colour and class* A fourth legacy of the slave system, perpetuated to some extent by the system of colonial government, is the ambivalent attitude of Negroes towards white people and their perception of their own social position. Stuart Hall, a West Indian sociologist, in an unpublished paper, has said graphically that a white person may be seen by West Indians as 'a distant friend and an intimate enemy'. He is an enemy in that he is a member of that group of people who preserved power and privilege very largely in their hands and who were the source of suffering and degradation for many coloured people, but he is an intimate enemy as his ancestors have been closely associated with the West Indies for four hundred years. He is a friend in that he has presided over a system of government, law, and education on which West Indians were heavily dependent for their advancement. In particular, there are those West Indians descended from house rather than field slaves who may also have served as their masters' concubines, who grow up in families where there has been a long and intimate association with white people; but these 'friendships' have necessarily been distant. Because of this background, in many of the relationships between

coloured West Indians and white people, there exists a mixture of deference, imitation, and resentment. The reactions of white people often do little to change this state of affairs.

Since slavery involved the treatment of Negroes as chattels and subhuman beings in their rights and duties, a caste-like system was established which associated blackness with slavery and inferiority and whiteness with power, influence, and high social status. These images, which were sometimes internalized by both white and coloured people, have been difficult for both to abandon, and many Negro people value lighter complexions highly. There is evidence of a distinct association between higher social class and status and lighter skin colour, and those coloured West Indians with lighter complexions, often the descendants of the children of plantation owners and slave women, may be both envied and resented by people with a darker skin colour. Few white people are aware of these distinctions; in Selvon's words, 'all you interested in that he black—to English people every black man look the same'.

Colonial legacies

A further extremely important influence in the lives of many West Indians has been the British colonial system which, to a large extent, transferred British customs and institutions to its subject countries. Since colonial administrators were drawn from the middle class, it was this style of life which served as a model for many West Indians. Furthermore, the isolation of the West Indies meant that this pattern became more fixed and more resistant to change than it did in Britain. Many West Indians were, therefore, brought up in a tradition which we would now regard as paternalistic, or even Victorian, in which Britain was seen as the mother, even the home country, with her sovereign commanding a degree of loyalty and respect which would now be unfamiliar to most English people.

The educational system, whose curriculum was, until recently, almost identical to that common in Britain, contributed to the development of this English identity and ensured that West Indian children might have quite a detailed knowledge of British history, geography, literature, and customs while being ignorant of their own environment.

The Christian Church is also influential in the West Indies and, especially amongst some working-class West Indians, a number of strict evangelical groups such as the Jehovah's Witnesses, the Seventh Day Adventists, and various Pentecostal sects are popular. Members of these sects do not consider great financial security a necessary condition of marriage, actively condemn common-law unions, and encourage a rather puritanical outlook. Until recently, most West Indians would consider themselves to be practising Christians to a much greater extent than the majority of the British population.

The intellectual and emotional focus of many of the West Indian islands, at least before gaining their independence was, therefore, on an English way of life, but one which was more familiar to the middle classes of earlier decades. In addition, for many people the wide discrepancies between their actual and their ideal way of life mean different models of parenthood and family life, all of which may be adopted by one person in the course of his lifetime. Relationships between poor working-class men and women, especially those which occur early, can often be expected to be unstable; and, in turn, the bonds between parents and children may not be clearly defined. The extended family provides some stability in this confusion; but since individuals may not remain dependent on it, and it is expected that they will do whatever they can to improve their position, with or without their family, this, too, is relatively weak.

The West Indian family in England

1 *Relationships between men and women* How far have these styles of life and attitudes continued in Britain? Partly because of the customs of their own social group, partly because they recognize that marriage is the most favoured kind of long-term union between English men and women, with the added advantage of tax incentives, and partly because of the fairly even number of men and women immigrants, many West Indian couples marry either before or after their emigration, sometimes causing the disruption of previous cohabitations. The opportunity for both men and women to earn removes the financial barrier to marriage; and this chance for men to support their families on a regular basis is potentially a stabilizing influence in West Indian family life. However, those who have been brought up in matriarchal families may have uncertain ideas about male and female roles, a confusion which is increased when they enter a society where these roles are still fairly clearly defined. Because of their upbringing, men may both resent and depend on women. Nor can they look forward to the day when, after marriage, they will be able to dominate their families, often because their economic plight demands that wives continue to work and contribute to the family income, thus maintaining some measure of independence.

Since some West Indian women have been brought up in a tradition where families, although idealistically patriarchal, were functionally matriarchal, they may be ambivalent about the ability of their menfolk to support them and thus contribute in no small way to their husband's dependence on them. While some women would like the opportunity of giving up work, others appreciate the independence their continued work gives them. In addition, partly because they are aware of the more equal relationship between husbands and wives in Britain, which does not depend entirely on the wife's contributing to the family income but which, nevertheless, expects a husband to play some part in the domestic affairs of the family, some West Indian women will resent their husbands' attempts to dominate their families and they will criticize them for not taking a greater share of the responsibility for their children's upbringing. Paradoxically, it is the more egalitarian partnership of cohabitation which more closely resembles an English marriage, rather than the relationship involving masculine dominance, typical of West Indian Christian marriage, which many couples have struggled to achieve. Whatever may be their feelings towards this kind of strict relationship, some West Indians will be bewildered and even shocked by the association in Britain between marriage and a man-woman relationship which is reminiscent of the cohabitation which they are so proud to have left behind.

Thus, in a number of subtle and complex ways, the relationship between West Indian men and women can be critically affected by their emigration, and their mutual ambivalence and hostility, more latent in the West Indies, may be spotlighted and provoked by the demands made on them in Britain. However, many men and women either welcome or adapt to these new demands. As the already fairly loose bonds between relatives are further weakened by migration, husbands and wives increasingly have to rely on each other for material support, the upbringing of children, and their emotional and social satisfaction; several studies have shown a greater degree of successful shared domesticity amongst West Indian couples in Britain than would have been expected before their migration. None the less, in some families the patriarchal role of the father is so well established and supported by religious beliefs that it goes virtually unchallenged by the mother, although it is doubtful whether it can survive the inevitable questioning and possible revolt of their children.

2 *The care of West Indian children in Britain* In the up-

bringing of their children, West Indian parents will naturally draw on their own experiences, and will expect obedience and tend to enforce discipline by external sanctions or threats which may seem severe to many English people but which reflect the West Indians' anxiety for their children to be seen as respectable. They do not all see the need to give children intellectual stimulation either by talking with them or providing play materials; and so, while valuing education highly, unwittingly they do not help their children to achieve the ambitions they have for them.

The pattern of life of many West Indian families in Britain is a complex mixture of working- and middle-class customs and attitudes. These subtleties are not apparent to most English people, who see West Indians as firmly belonging to the working class, a quite different estimation to that of the West Indians themselves. This precarious social status is likely to make West Indians anxious about any aspects of their behaviour which might threaten it even further. In particular, their anxiety may influence their feelings towards their illegitimate children.

The somewhat uncertain structure of West Indian family life in Britain, together with the sometimes confused relationships between men and women and the continuing importance attached to proofs of female fertility and motherhood, is likely to contribute to a fair number of illegitimate births and single parent families. However, many parents are aware of both the greater social disgrace of such a predicament in Britain, as well as the great difficulty in caring for an illegitimate child in a country where its female relatives could all be expected to go out to work and where its reception into care would be strongly resisted by many social work agencies; they will, therefore, be more than usually anxious to protect their daughters from such a plight, possibly bringing fiercer sanctions on a girl who becomes illegitimately pregnant than would be customary in the West Indies. Nevertheless, after facing initial anger and rejection, the erring daughter is often reconciled to her family when the child is born, and attempts are made to arrange some kind of care for the infant.

Various factors in Britain, including the widespread disapproval of illegitimacy and the likelihood that many fathers of illegitimate children may now be married, with prior responsibilities towards their wives and legitimate children, may result in an increasing number of women who can expect little support from the fathers of their children or their other relatives. Influenced by the custom in the West Indies, they recognize that little apart from emnity is likely to be achieved by taking out affiliation orders and so strongly resist the pressures on them from English social workers to do this. By remaining on good terms with their children's fathers they hope to improve their chances of receiving some maintenance from them. Fitzherbert (1967) has described how very pliable the relationship between a West Indian father and his illegitimate child can be, ranging from a recognition of absolute responsibility to complete irresponsibility, depending very much on the man's relationship with the child's mother and his economic position and varying from time to time according to his circumstances.

The plight of the single-parent West Indian family, living on the edge of poverty and heavily dependent on the services of child minders, whose standard of care is variable, has already been described; it is well recognized that children living in these circumstances may be seriously retarded, emotionally and educationally. However, M. Pollak (1970) produces some disturbing evidence that some West Indian three-year-olds living with both parents in relatively stable family units are more backward than similarly placed white English children, especially in their language and social development.

It is difficult to make reliable comparisons when testing children from different cultural or ethnic backgrounds. Nevertheless, given the extra difficulties under which the

West Indian families in this study were labouring, it is not surprising that their young children showed more evidence of handicap than did their white peers. Pollak found that the West Indian families lived in poorer, more over-crowded, more expensive accommodation than white families; that far more West Indian mothers worked full time, placing their children more frequently in the care of unofficial and cheaper daily minders. Many more West Indian than white children had been cared for by several daily minders. Nearly three-quarters of the West Indian children had stepfathers; and while this could mean some family tensions, the most serious consequence seemed to be the need for one or both parents to contribute to the keep of other children living in the West Indies, thus exacerbating the families' already acute financial struggle, a major part of which fell on the shoulders of the mothers. Inevitably, the quality of mothering available to the children living with their parents was severely affected and they had little opportunity of stimulation, play, and social contact. Other studies, including one by Hood *et al.* (1970), have come to similar conclusions.

The outlook for the emotional and educational development of children living in these circumstances is bleak. Although they may be helped by early compensatory education, it is more important for their parents to have some relief from the acute financial pressures on them. We also need to bear in mind the fact that some young West Indian women, although valuing the state of motherhood, may have little inclination for the everyday practical care of their children, or experience of this, since in the West Indies it may largely be left in the hands of their older female relatives; it is these women who provide the emotional warmth and stimulation which children need, while their young mothers play a more paternal role in their financial support. The average daily minder is proving to be a poor substitute for the West Indian aunt or grandmother, a fact that may not always be apparent to women who have little conception of Western standards of child care. We have to think seriously about the need to provide high-quality substitute day care for children whose mothers go out to work.

3 *Flexibility and adaptation* Social workers may see in some West Indian families a pattern of disrupted or unstable relationships which they would expect to have disastrous consequences in most English families. However, following a pattern of accommodation and adaptation common in the West Indies, many families appear to absorb these difficulties and, perhaps as a direct consequence, their attitudes towards parental and other responsibilities may be varied and flexible. A man may be an excellent stepfather but show little concern for his own illegitimate children; a woman may vow to have nothing to do with a relative whom she believes has shamed her but ultimately does all she can to help in a crisis. It is helpful, therefore, not to expect consistency in the acceptance of certain responsibilities, nor to despair when faced with sudden, apparently serious changes in relationships. At the same time, however, the various pressures on West Indians in Britain make it likely that family problems assume more serious proportions than they might have done before immigration.

4 *Relationships with English people* Added to these strains on an already rather insecure family structure, many West Indian immigrants experience a special sense of disillusionment and disappointment in their expectations of Britain as the mother country. A rather hazy and old-fashioned image of England has been a part of their childhood and they are shocked to find that this image if far from the reality of life in the UK. Not only are their values seen as quaint and outdated, but they find they are unwelcome strangers about whom most people know nothing. In no sense does the 'mother' country welcome her

distant children, rather she regards them as inferior and makes few distinctions as to their colour or class. Faced with this rebuff, many West Indians are confused and bitter. Having regarded themselves in all important respects as English, they have few alternative cultural or national groups into which they can withdraw for security and protection. Partly as a result of this isolation and the many rebuffs they experience, some younger West Indians are now finding security in movements which emphasize Black Power ideals and the need for coloured people to be independent and self-supporting. These organizations are often regarded with horror by the older, more conservative West Indians.

West Indians' relationships with their white neighbours, frequently working-class people, are likely to be strained because each group may regard the other as inferior. Equally difficult in different ways are their more formal relationships with middle-class people such as teachers and social workers, who are confused by the paradox of the resourcefulness of West Indian immigrants and the kind of dependence on representatives of the social services that they may at times reveal. These representatives feel uneasy when they realize that partly because of the association in the immigrant's minds of white officialdom with authority and the command of resources, and partly because of the immigrants' lack of knowledge about the function of the social services, they are being invested with more power that they really have. Requests that the 'government' should care for erring children and change their behaviour, and that teachers should 'school a child well to be a lawyer', can arouse irritation and resentment, just as failure to comply with these requests leaves many West Indians upset and confused. In particular, they resent refusals of help which they see as essential to maintaining a pattern of life important for economic or social reasons and which, in the West Indies, would be provided by the extended family. However, for a number of reasons, including the ignorance and confusion of some officials, their own emotional reserve, and the deference, albeit sometimes resentful, with which they are treated by West Indians and which inhibits any expression of feeling or opinion, there is frequently very little explanation of the background of requests or the reasons for their refusal.

Another paradox which puzzles and irritates English people is the gap—which has its roots deep in the social system of the West Indies—between the life values professed as ideal by many West Indians and the life they actually live. Although this gap usually narrows after immigration, some English people may still detect a failure to abide by the Christian virtues that many West Indians strongly profess, a discrepancy between middle-class ideals and their actual social status, and a reluctance to make any allowance, at least verbally, for behaviour in others in which they may themselves have indulged at an earlier stage in their life. This double standard, which can involve some self-deception, combined with the attitudes of West Indians towards people in authority, makes it difficult for them to be open about their circumstances and feelings and even to face up to some of the realities of life. Misunderstandings multiply, and West Indians are often seen in an unsympathetic light. As they come to perceive some of their ideals and aspirations as a source of bitter frustration as well as inspiration, it will probably be even harder for West Indians to discuss their ambitions and their circumstances. Social workers need to be most sensitive to the reasons for these different standards and the frequent disappointments that accompany them.

5   *Use of social services*   For all these reasons, the West Indian immigrant, who had expected to fit easily into the English way of life, occupies a particularly vulnerable position in British society. Above all, many West Indians lack the support of a stable extended family and the security of a cultural or national identity which are so

important to first-generation immigrants. Not surprisingly, therefore, they make proportionately more demands on the social services, particularly children's services, than any other coloured immigrant group.

Many single West Indian mothers would be most un-happy to stay at home to live on Supplementary Benefits. Not only would this leave them in a very isolated position, but it is so contrary to the pattern of life with which they are familiar that they may actually feel guilty if they are not able to earn money to buy their children extra luxuries. Some women may also be anxious to take training courses which, by ensuring them a good wage and high social status in the long run, will mean they are in an excellent position to support their families. Added to this is the pressure on some West Indian mothers to contribute to the upkeep of their children in the West Indies. When West Indians are unable to find day-minding facilities which they can afford, they turn, with little hesitation, towards the Child Care services, often believing that a child placed in residential care will have an excellent boarding educa-tion with the special advantage of being brought up by white people. They may show little awareness of the trauma experienced by many children who are separated from their parents, or anxiety lest their children, after growing up in a very different environment, should be confused or resentful when they return home either at secondary school age or when they are able to go out to work.

This view of residential child care as a golden oppor-tunity is quite at variance with the views held by most social workers. They are aware of the pressures on resi-dential services, their shortcomings, and some of the special problems of identification faced by West Indian children cared for by white people, as well as the cardinal principle that young children should only be separated from their parents only if there is absolutely no alternative. Such a discrepancy in outlook is bound to lead to misunderstandings and conflict. These cannot always be removed by discussion and explanation when the beliefs held by each party are so very deep-rooted and divergent, and make the sharing of opinions difficult. None the less, social workers need to show that they are aware of the special dilemma of the West Indian family, to explain their own views, and to listen to those of their clients, partly because this can lead to some mutual and helpful modifications, but also because a failure to do this results in continued confusion and the alienation of West Indians and the social services from each other.

Fitzherbert (1967) has argued that because of the misunderstandings West Indians have about the Child Care service, the special disadvantages suffered by coloured children in care, and the ability of many parents to find alternative care for their children, Child Care Officers should resist particularly strongly their requests for reception into care. However, this view does not sufficiently take into account the weakening bonds of the West Indian extended family in Britain or the very poor quality of daily or foster care on which many immigrants have to depend. Holman's studies (1968) show clearly that refusal to admit to care does not necessarily prevent problems for the child and his family, and may in some cases lead to serious difficulties.

The extent to which the social services should be adapted to meet the needs of particular minority groups will be discussed in a later section. However, it is useful here to ask how worth-while it is to expect West Indian mothers and those who share their predicament to adopt a way of life which they regard as unnatural and not in the interests of themselves or their children. Staying at home may involve an intolerable degree of isolation and poverty; going out to work may mean making hopelessly unsatisfactory arrangements for their children. Bearing in mind the disadvantages of residential care and the lack of substitute care with relatives, local authorities need to consider whether, in the absence of sufficient day nurseries, they should make financial contributions towards other forms of care. This might sometimes involve an allowance, making it possible for a mother to place her child with a more adequate and expensive daily minder, or alternatively it could mean financing places in playgroups on a far more lavish scale than is usually the practice, both for children living with their parents continuously and for those who are cared for during the day outside their home and in a poor environment. Such policies obviously beg questions about financing services which may sometimes be of a rather lower standard than those sponsored by local authorities. But in the absence of fully adequate facilities, a failure to do this means that a large number of children, including many West Indians, will be cared for in the most unsatisfactory circumstances during one of the most important and most impressionable periods of their life.

Children of mixed racial background

Since the majority of children with a mixed racial background are born to West Indian and English parents, it is reasonable to include them in this section. Perhaps the most striking and well-known fact about these children is their great over-representation in residential care. Although we do not know what percentage these children form of all the children with mixed racial background, some studies have indicated that when they are born into an insecure environment, which may include parents who are unmarried or separated and the objects of social disapproval, they run a great risk of going into care and even of being totally rejected. A Barnardo's working committee (1966) reported that in 1965 slightly over 20 per cent of children in their homes were coloured, including those children of mixed racial background. However, nearly 70 per cent of these children had West Indian (by far the largest group),

Indian, or Pakistani fathers and English mothers. A substantial proportion had little or no contact with their parents. Even more disturbingly, Foren and Batta (1970) found that in Bradford, between 1966 and 1969, children of mixed racial parentage had a very much greater chance of going into care than either white or fully coloured children. One child in twelve born of mixed parentage was received into care before the age of five, compared with less than one in every hundred white or fully coloured children. Furthermore, a substantial number of these children had been deserted or abandoned by their mothers, nearly all came into care before they were five years old, and many stayed in care for long periods.

It is only possible to speculate about the circumstances which contribute to the vulnerability of these children. There is some evidence that many of the white girls who form relationships with coloured men have been rejected by their husbands or boy-friends and already have children. Some, too, are themselves immigrants from Scotland or Ireland and so, isolated from their families, feel an affinity with people who share their position. It has also been observed that in an atmosphere where coloured people are regarded as inferior there is a chance that some white women, who are themselves regarded as inadequate by white men, may seek the company of coloured men; some of these men, because of their loneliness or a tendency to see a white girl-friend as a status symbol, fail to realize that these girls will probably not be satisfactory companions or wives. When children are born to these unions, their mothers are especially unlikely to be able to care for them adequately, and there is a tendency for them to prefer their white children. However, there is some evidence that coloured fathers show a closer interest in these children and a greater willingness to visit than white fathers in similar circumstances. Further difficulties are caused by relatives refusing to have anything to do with someone who has a half-coloured child, and by the prevailing myth that children of 'mixed blood' are in some way inherently inferior and likely to exhibit the worst attributes of both their mothers and fathers.

It would be wrong to assume that social workers share this myth; but, none the less, many regard children of mixed racial backgrounds as presenting some of their most difficult problems. While this may well be true, it is important to realize that although there is some overlap between the difficulties arising from a child's racial background and the difficulties arising from his rejection, it is the rejection of the child by its mother and, in turn, her rejection by her family which lie at the root of the problems with which social workers have to deal. In addition, the possession of a coloured child may be the symptom rather than the cause of the personal unhappiness and inadequacy which contribute to a woman's failure as a mother. Social workers have much experience of these difficulties, and if they can focus their work in this direction, preferably before a child is born, some of the fatalism which so often surrounds discussion of the future of children of mixed parentage could disappear. It is also significant that until recently, partly because prospective adoptive parents were not asked whether they would like a child of mixed racial background, such children had little chance of being adopted. Some recent studies, in particular that by Raynor (1971), indicate that there is a demand for these children, although their placement and supervision may need to be most skilfully carried out.

Chapter 4 described briefly some of the problems of those children of mixed racial background who remain with their parents. They may have a special need to talk about the conflicting pull they feel on their loyalties within their families as well as the peculiar attitudes towards their background which they will almost certainly encounter. Instead of this opportunity for discussion there is often a collusive silence amongst the children, their parents, teachers, and social workers; this reflects the embarrassed curiosity, and even shame, with which the children of mixed racial background are sometimes regarded and which contributes to their withdrawal and alienation.

As one of the groups most vulnerable to rejection and deprivation, children of mixed racial background may need very special attention and care. The treatment they receive will be the surest reflection of the feelings of white and coloured people about their relationships with each other.

Pakistanis in Britain

Pakistanis make up the smallest of the major immigrant groups from the New Commonwealth. In 1966 it was estimated that, excluding white Pakistanis, there were less than 200,000 people in Britain who had themselves been born in Pakistan or whose parents had been. Pakistanis have settled mainly in the south-east of England, Yorkshire, and the West Midlands, where they have been employed in large numbers in some of the least attractive industries, particularly those producing cloth and rubber. However, since they are a highly mobile group and move readily from town to town in search of work, small settlements of Pakistani immigrants and their families can be found in many large towns where there is a demand for labour. Until very recently Pakistani immigrants were mainly young men, but increasingly wives and children are coming to England as their menfolk become more established and prosperous and as the various immigration Acts make it more difficult for resident immigrants to travel freely between England and Pakistan, thus making contact with absent families more and more uncertain. However, in 1966 there was still a large imbalance between the sexes, and in some areas men outnumbered women by nearly ten to one. Since there is so far little inter-marriage between Pakistanis and English women, many

143

of those men who intend to stay in England, at least for some years, return to Pakistan to be married, and at some stage bring their wives to Britain. Some people believe that the reunion and settlement of Pakistani families is only just beginning and that their numbers will increase substantially in the next few years. In some towns many families have already been reunited.

Social, political, and religious traditions

So far very little has been written about the settlement of Pakistanis in Britain and there are no detailed accounts of the life of Pakistani families before their immigration. We must, therefore, depend on the various accounts of the immigrants themselves and some rather general observations of people who have made some local studies of Pakistani settlements in Britain or who have been concerned with them. What is clear, however, is that as with all immigrant groups, care should be taken not to generalize about the beliefs and customs of people who come from widely differing parts of Pakistan, where different languages are spoken, and who may belong to a variety of social groups. Although the great majority of Pakistanis are Moslems, their devotion to Islam, while it provides some common background and sometimes a unifying influence, is likely to be interpreted in different ways and with greater or less strictness according to the particular circumstances and inclinations of individuals. Amongst Moslems who count themselves as orthodox, just as with Christians, it is possible to identify wide variations of belief and custom, and it is, therefore, wise not to make any assumptions about religious practice and to take care to understand the different meanings Islam has for individual Pakistanis. A minority of Christian Pakistanis have also settled in Britain, and although their style of life often reflects Islamic traditions, they would be most offended to be thought of as Moslems. Their position in society is difficult, since they are accepted neither by their Moslem compatriots nor by their fellow Christians who are natives of Britain.

It is not always appreciated that East and West Pakistan are over a thousand miles apart and have little in common apart from some religious traditions. Pakistanis' awareness of belonging to the same nation has long been compromised by serious rivalries between the East and West, with the West being seen as more prosperous with too little sense of responsibility or obligation towards the East which has now claimed independence as the state of Bangla Desh. Geographically, and in many other ways, the main areas of emigration differ sharply from each other. In the West, the Mirpur area which borders on Kashmir, the Campbellpore area of the North West Frontier Province, and the border areas of the Punjab are dry, mountainous regions, providing only a bare subsistence for the peasants who farm there. The most common language is Punjabi and its various dialects, although Urdu is understood by the more educated people. Emigrants from East Pakistan come mainly from the Sylhet region and the maritime provinces around the Bay of Bengal. Potentially this is a fertile region, but its violent tropical climate threatens the security of the inhabitants and contributes to numerous natural disasters, the greatest being the flood disaster in 1970 in which it is estimated that between two and five hundred thousand people died and many thousands more were made homeless. Bengali is the most widely spoken language in East Pakistan.

In both East and West Pakistan there have been substantial movements of population as a result of the 1947 partition between India and Pakistan which established the latter as an Islamic state for the Moslem population of the Indian sub-continent. Millions more Pakistanis became refugees in the tragic aftermath of the civil war between East and West Pakistan in 1971. Large parts of the population have, therefore, had direct experience of the hardship of resettlement and the agonies of political upheaval.

In both East and West Pakistan there is substantial illiteracy, and this is naturally reflected amongst the immigrants in Britain.

The majority of emigrants from Pakistan, who represent only a tiny minority of the total population, belong to peasant farming families whose poverty has bred a tradition whereby their younger male members were sent abroad, or to industrial regions, or to sea to earn money for the rest of the family. Many Pakistanis have already some experience of urban industrial life before coming to Britain. Members of an extended family, who might make up a whole village, pool their resources to finance this migration; and it is understood that once one family member is established, he will not only send money back to his family, but will also sponsor other immigrants by helping with their fares and their settlement. This system of sponsorship provides immigrants with some security, but it also creates strong bonds of obligation between members of the same village or extended family from which a migrant may never be able to release himself. It also contributes to petty jealousies and rivalries amongst different regional groups, which makes it hard for Pakistani immigrants to see themselves as a group of people with common interests and needs and for recognized leaders to emerge because political loyalties run parallel to kinship and village loyalties.

Settlement in Britain

The migration of men without their families was the most usual pattern for Pakistanis in Britain until the mid-1960s. The immigrants were, to a large extent, voluntary exiles in a foreign country whose aim in life was to earn as much as possible, as quickly as possible, however much personal discomfort and unhappiness this involved. Many of them hoped, and continue to hope that by acquiring wealth in Britain they would be able to establish themselves successfully when they returned home in a way that is usually impossible for those without family connections and capital. They might return for a holiday in Pakistan after a few years in Britain, or their places might be taken by other family members, thus establishing an almost continuous rota of migration. These immigrants' attention was directed towards Pakistan, and they were isolated, partly by choice, into tight-knit village and family groups, making little impact on British society and asking nothing from it, except to be allowed to work and save. Even when these groups of young male migrants contained school-aged boys, who were waiting to join their older relations in employment and who had little in the way of a home life, they were largely self-sufficient and made few calls on the social services, although the conditions in which they were either prepared or forced to live were the source of some concern. The single male immigrant, with few social connections, who lives in a lodging-house, and who fills as many hours as possible with work faces a bleak existence. His way of life is more likely to attract unfavourable attention since without the bonds of a family or close friends, there are fewer constraints on his behaviour.

The arrival of Pakistani wives and children substantially changes this pattern of life. The expense involved usually means that the families concerned have at least half acknowledged that their future, anyway for the next decade or so, lies in Britain. This can represent a major shift of focus in a family's aspirations. In meeting their responsibilities to provide suitable accommodation for their families and education for their children, many Pakistani men are brought into closer contact with the wider community than was customary in their 'bachelor' existence; some degree of adaptation to British society can, therefore, be expected. However, to some extent, the arrival of families is also an isolating factor. This is partly because family life now provides a comfortable alternative to accommodation to English customs and institutions, and the presence of women and children reinforces the obligations Moslems feel to provide an appropriate environment for the practice of Islamic religious and social ideals. Various business enterprises, at which Pakistanis excel, and which cater primarily for their own community, also tend to make them relatively self-sufficient. Within such a context Rose (1969) detects the beginnings of some fusion amongst the different groups of Pakistanis, who are beginning to recognize the common needs of their families.

Islamic social and religious influences

What then are the cultural and religious traditions of which social workers need to be aware when they meet Pakistani families? To a large extent these traditions are inseparable because Islam, more than most religions, lays down a code of moral and social conduct which greatly influences the day-to-day life of its faithful. Laws regarding marriage, inheritance, and family responsibilities are rooted in Islamic tradition, as revealed either in the Koran, the Moslem holy book, or in canon law. These traditions are often further sanctioned by the civil law of the Islamic states, of which Pakistan is the largest. In this way, the life of a Pakistani—or, indeed, of any citizen of a Moslem state, even if he is not religious himself—is much influenced by customs and laws which have their origin in the religious and social teachings of Islam. In some cases, too, these teachings have been misinterpreted, and there have developed cultural traditions which, although identified with the Moslem way of life, do not in fact accord to strict Islamic belief.

Islam literally means submission to the Will of Allah, a compassionate and merciful God who is fundamentally the God of Christianity and Judaism and whose major prophet was Mohammed. It is a monotheistic religion, and its links with Christianity and Judaism are clearly shown in the Koran. However, some Moslems regard themselves as God's people, chosen above all others, with a unique heritage to preserve and pass on; they, therefore, feel superior to non-Moslems and are conscious of their separate identity. The main religious institutions of Islam involve saying prayers, if possible five times a day, fasting for one month a year during Ramadhan from dawn to sunset, giving of alms, and making the pilgrimage to Mecca for those who can afford it. Moslems are also forbidden to eat any pig meat or to drink alcohol. Like orthodox Jews, they are bound to eat only the meat of animals that have been slaughtered by bleeding, and this makes many English tinned foods and meat products unacceptable. Taboos of this kind lead many Pakistanis to be very anxious about eating any food that has been prepared by English people. Clearly this can present problems for men who are expected to eat in factory canteens and children who have their lunch at school. These religious customs may be more or less strictly interpreted, but there are Islamic social traditions which greatly influence family life.

1   *Family responsibilities*   First and foremost, these traditions emphasize the responsibilities of family members for each other. The family network is a wide one and includes, in particular, male relatives and their descendants. Unmarried women and girls are also the responsibility of the family until they marry, at which point they move into the orbit and protection of their husbands' families. Although polygamy is tolerated, it is not encouraged, and very few Moslems have more than one wife. The able-bodied members of the family support the aged, children, widows, and those who, for a variety of reasons, are not able to support themselves. In Pakistan the conduct of family affairs, the farming of land, and the sharing of resources will be very much a matter of joint

negotiation; members of a family group will be conscious not of their own individuality, but of their dependence on and loyalty to their relatives, and will regard life outside this context as impossible and meaningless. Such an environment provides the possibility of great affection and approval for the individual, but it also greatly multiplies the opportunities for disapproval and family disgrace.

2 *The position of women*

> To treat purda as a religious injunction is to miss the point, for it is much more than that. It is an integral part of social organisation and is closely interrelated with roles and relationships, allocation of rights and duties within the family and with the kinship system in regard to descent, inheritance and succession; it is one of the most important means of expressing and acquiring prestige (Dahya, 1965, pp. 316-17).

The position of women in Moslem families is complex. Although men and women are accepted as equal in Moslem law and various provisions through inheritance and marriage settlements ensure the financial security of women, in many Moslem families it is the men who play the dominant and public roles. Most women expect to have their marriages arranged for them, and they are expected to behave submissively and modestly. In some families this involves their seclusion from all males apart from certain relatives, and some women will veil their faces in public. Women and children will often eat separately from men and only after they have served them their meals. While a man's social life is often conducted outside the home, a woman is usually expected to remain within the confines of her family on whom she is dependent for companionship and social contact. This chance of companionship may be greatly reduced when the Pakistani woman emigrates, and she may find herself isolated and lonely in Britain, cut off from the rest of the community by both custom and language and without the support of the extended family. Since Pakistanis tend to confine their friendships and social contacts to the family circle, a woman without relatives in Britain can be very lonely and have little opportunity to meet other Pakistani women who are similarly placed. Unless she has some opportunity to learn English, she can lead a solitary life.

It is not always clear what influence a woman exerts within her own family. Certainly when a young girl marries and goes to live with her husband's family she is expected to be respectful and obedient and not to challenge her husband's relationships with his own parents or kinsmen. From birth she will have been brought up to value the only role acceptable for women, that of a devoted wife and mother, and her chief aspiration is likely to be the perfect fulfillment of this role. Although her life may seem very restricted by European standards, she can expect the security of the support of her male relatives, particularly her husband and brothers, who take their family responsibilities very seriously and who are most unlikely to desert her. Indeed the high value placed by Pakistani men on family life potentially puts women in a position of some honour and respect within that context.

Although a Pakistani woman will have some influence over her young children it is not until she is older and one of the senior members of the family that she will have much voice in its affairs. Even then, this influence will be exerted in private, and in public she will continue to play the role of a dutiful and submissive wife. It would be most unwise, therefore, to try to draw a woman into a public discussion or argument about family affairs. When it is necessary for young Pakistani women to play a part in making decisions, their inexperience of this can make them appear passive and rather helpless. They need a great deal of patient support before they are able to take on a more active role.

3 *The upbringing of children* Young children are looked

after by their mothers and female relatives, and since it is most unusual for Pakistani women to work, these children are constantly surrounded by people who care for them; thus they have the opportunity of imitative play—although they may have few toys—and joining in household tasks. As boys grow older they move more under the influence of their fathers and male relatives, and from the age of seven, in theory at least, their fathers are seen as having chief responsibility for them. Boys are usually valued more than girls largely because of the positive economic contribution they will be able to make to the family fortunes, while girls are a drain on the family income because of the dowry which must be provided on their marriage. Some people see the relationship between father and son as being the strongest and most influential in Pakistani family life.

As girls grow up, they are increasingly secluded from contact with males, particularly after they reach the age of puberty. As members of an extended family with clearly defined responsibilities, children are expected to be respectful and obedient, even subservient, to their elders, and girls must avoid any behaviour which makes them less attractive as prospective brides. Any kind of liaison with the opposite sex, however innocent, is frowned on and a sexual misadventure severely punished. If possible, such behaviour will be hushed up completely, as a girl with sexual experience is highly unlikely to be thought suitable as a wife. While fairly tolerant of their son's misdemeanours, parents are very careful about the upbringing of their daughters and anxious to discourage any independent behaviour or attitudes which might make it difficult for a girl to settle in and be accepted by her future husband's family. Recognizing the humble position a young wife occupies on her marriage, they want her to be prepared for this throughout her childhood. Both boys and girls are likely to receive fairly extensive instruction in the Islamic faith, and their mothers, especially, are said to encourage this, as they see it as a way of preserving their children's respect for the family and bond with their parents. Mosques have been established in Britain, and some Moslem children attend special religious instruction classes.

This sense of order in family life, of fixed rights and obligations, and of an established hierarchy, plus the influence of Islam, emphasizing submission to the Divine Will, may inhibit what Europeans would see as the free and normal expression of feeling. Certainly affection, particularly between the opposite sexes, is not displayed in public. Nor is there usually public expression of family conflict or ill-feeling between relatives. This makes it hard for Pakistanis and English people, each inhibited in their own ways, to communicate with each other; many English people find Pakistanis inscrutable and are unable to gauge their attitudes or feelings. In many cases this difficulty arises because social workers have been unable to recognize the different ways people communicate their anxiety or hostility. For Pakistanis it is common to exhibit rather withdrawn behaviour, and although they may have strong views about many aspects of the English way of life, they are unlikely to discuss them freely with English people until they feel at ease with them. Opportunities for misunderstandings and failure of communication multiply especially when social workers, feeling uneasy at their first contact, identify these problems as an insuperable cultural barrier and fail to persevere in developing relationships with Pakistani clients as they would do with more familiar, but equally distant, native clients.

4 *The tradition of mutual self-help* The extent to which these traditions and beliefs are established in a family will, of course, depend on its length of settlement in Britain and its social class. In general, the higher and more educated groups will interpret Islamic traditions more liberally. However, since many immigrants are peasants

with a tradition of conservatism, it is likely that they will adhere fairly strictly, at least in principle, to most of the customs described. So far their family solidarity has prevented their making many calls on the social services; and most families, even though they may be far more fragmented than in Pakistan, have kept alive their tradition of self-help. There are established methods of solving family disputes, including marital difficulties and the custody of children, and although these settlements may sometimes seem harsh to English people, they are usually the preferred solution of Pakistanis. The rare occasions when social workers are asked to intervene in family affairs usually indicate very serious discord or difficulty, or an unusual degree of separation of the family concerned from its wider family network, which therefore, makes them dependent, like English families, on substitute methods of help. In such situations social workers need to discover why there has been a request for help outside the family and whether the problem can more appropriately be solved outside the family context. In cases of extreme difficulty, such as the illegitimate pregnancy of a young woman, her family may well feel unable to give her any help at all, and she may even need some protection from their wrath. However, in less acute cases, partly depending on the length of the family's settlement in Britain and its degree of independence, it may be more helpful to try to solve problems within the family's own confines, possibly, if the family is agreeable, with the assistance of the local Pakistani community. Issues such as confidentiality and personal self-determination need to be interpreted in the light of what would be usual and accepted by the individual or family concerned; this may differ considerably from the expectations of English people used to living in greater isolation and privacy. The implications of social work with extended families will be more fully discussed in the next chapter.

Social work involvement

Many social workers now find that the extent to which they are concerned with Pakistani families depends largely on their own initiative. Some believe they have an important role to play as 'bridge people' or interpreters of the various social services, particularly those concerned with health and education. Others are especially concerned by the isolation of many Pakistani women and its implications for the upbringing of their children. They believe it is important to reach out to them by providing English classes and other opportunities for social contact. Provided that these arrangements do not involve Pakistani women in too great or sudden exposure to outside influences, they are usually welcomed by the women and their families, although it may take some time before confidence is established between them and their teachers and social workers. To accomplish this, the social worker usually visits families, meeting the various members. Attempts at contact by letter are usually unsuccessful, partly because of illiteracy, but also because this kind of communication is frequently misunderstood and mistrusted.

1 *Some current anxieties*   Whatever the nature of their contact with Pakistani families, English social workers are likely to be puzzled and disturbed by two things. In the first place, they may be distressed by the subordinate position of women, amazed by the women's apparent acceptance of it, and horrified by their willingness to have their husbands selected for them. The position of women in Moslem society is a much disputed subject, and many attempts have been made in Pakistan and elsewhere to improve their position and to establish some of their rights and independence. These attempts have been partially successful, although they meet with opposition from orthodox men and women. While it is easy to understand the basis for men's objections to greater female independence, the attitude of women is more complex.

Even though many of the constraints on their freedom may give rise to resentment, women also find security in their fixed position and in their dependence on their families, which protects them from major responsibility in family affairs and decision-making about their own future when they may feel they have very little basis on which to form sound opinions.

This sense of dependence is heightened by migration, and many Pakistani women would be appalled if they had to take greater personal responsibility for their own lives and their children's. They are often shocked by the much freer relationships between English men and women, and regard these as directly responsible for the weak family structure which they see everywhere in Britain. On the other hand, they are often desperately lonely and isolated and fearful for their future as their children grow up. Their wish for more independence will, therefore, be an ambivalent one, and social workers need to recognize that these women will only move slowly towards achieving any measure of independence because this involves a change in traditions which have been established for centuries. It is hard for social workers to accept customs about which they may feel sensitive and which are currently the focus of public concern or dispute; and although self-evident, it still needs to be emphasized that it can be quite inappropriate and unethical for social workers to seek to impose their own traditions and beliefs on immigrants. Nevertheless, this is a contentious issue which will be more fully considered in chapter 6.

Second, social workers are quite likely to be confused by their relationships with Pakistanis who treat authority figures with a distant respect and deference which mask their real feeling. As a consequence, social workers sometimes feel that Pakistanis are telling them only what they think their listeners want to hear. This behaviour is partly due to traditions about the expression of feelings, which have already been described. It is also connected with an

initial distrust that many Pakistanis feel towards outsiders, particularly non-Moslems, who may be seen as part
of the long train of officials who have some power over
their lives, although totally alienated from them, and who
need to be placated, even to the extent of being offered
bribes. This sense of distance may be heightened if the
social worker is a woman working with male Pakistanis
as she would be almost bound to do in family affairs.
Equally many Pakistanis would be shocked and insulted
if a male social worker tried to make contact with their
women or if the women were asked to visit an office where
they would run the risk of being seen by men.

Social workers also find their relationships with Pakistanis complicated when they think their clients are pas-
sively accepting problems and circumstances which would
be the cause of protest and distress to most English people.
This attitude needs to be understood in its religious context, and while it sometimes provides some temporary
protection for the individuals who adopt it, it does not
necessarily mean they will do nothing to alleviate their
position. Their migration bears testimony to this.

None of these difficulties is insurmountable, although
social workers may have to spend more time than usual
in establishing relationships, which may often seem quite
social, with Pakistani families. Once these relationships
have been established, it is often appropriate to draw
attention to some of the problems of communication that
exist and attempt to discuss these quite openly.

2 *Future contact* Whether social workers' contact with
Pakistani families remains largely peripheral will depend
partly on how far they decide to involve themselves in
crisis situations or to establish services which aim to
provide links between Pakistanis and the wider community. It will also depend on the extent to which Pakistani families remain largely self-sufficient and develop as a
recognized national group or community based on Islamic

ideals, with a separate identity and with its own methods of self-help.

Pakistani settlement and adaptation

At the moment, the evidence of adaptation or withdrawal and isolation is conflicting. On the one hand, Pakistanis are showing themselves to be largely independent of English institutions, anxious to avoid competition with English people, and eager to be left in peace to establish themselves economically. Language difficulties are also a serious barrier to communication. Furthermore, although they recognize themselves as members of the Commonwealth, this is nothing like as important to Pakistanis as it is to West Indians. Pakistanis have their own nation, and its religious and cultural traditions, particularly for the poorer people, have prevented any wholesale adoption of English customs and values. Indeed, as a minority subject to British rule for generations, many Moslems feel some hostility to English culture and are secure in their belief of the superiority of their own values. Like many migrants, most Pakistanis would say, if asked, that they intended eventually to return to their homelands, and it is not uncommon for their sons and daughters to return to Pakistan to marry. Indeed, there is some feeling that girls who spend their adolescence in England may run such risks of compromising themselves that they will not be seen as suitable brides by other Pakistanis. Most Moslem parents would be unhappy if their children married English people.

The self-sufficiency and isolation of Pakistanis is viewed with some ambivalence by the rest of the community, being both the source of admiration and some relief as well as the focus of suspicion and hostility, particularly from those who are the immediate neighbours of Pakistanis. The origin of these attitudes, which are similar to those displayed towards foreign Jewish immigrants in the early part of the century, is not clear. Partly they seem to emerge when a deprived community is seeking a scapegoat for its miseries and finds a group about which so little is known and which is so isolated that it is possible for fantastic stories about it to be invented and believed. A scapegoat also needs to be a 'safegoat' in that it will not retaliate, and certainly the majority of Pakistanis respond to antagonism by further withdrawal, although sometimes reserving the right to protect themselves. Their self-sufficiency, isolation, and commitment to their culture are, therefore, increased and the likelihood of consultation with native social workers reduced.

On the other hand, however, there are pressures for Pakistanis to make some adaptation to the demands of British society. In particular, as the case of the Khan family shows, the education of their children will bring them into contact, and sometimes conflict, with English values and institutions. Even if Pakistani children are able to live some kind of dual life, adapting themselves to both home and school, their education cannot fail to have an impact on their families and present them with choices in their social and religious customs. In addition, it is likely that the political and economic upheavals in Pakistan and Bangla Desh will encourage the permanent settlement of their emigrants. Many Pakistanis are aware that by migration they have immeasurably improved their own social standing in their family and village group and have, to a large extent, escaped the constraints that a strict social hierarchy would impose on their progress in Pakistan. The longer they are in Britain and the more their relatives come to join them, the less likely it is that their permanent return to Pakistan becomes a real possibility.

After some years, in the absence of a national identity, religious traditions may become more important, and it is possible that the children of Pakistani immigrants may grow up to see themselves as an Anglo-Islamic community, whose chief loyalty is to Britain, but whose way of life is influenced to some extent by Moslem ideals. How widely they will be distributed amongst the different social and occupational groups is not clear, since the great majority of Pakistani children are only just beginning school; we do not know what their aspirations will be, nor how far it will be possible for them to be realized, although the evidence from the experiences of other coloured immigrant groups, particularly the West Indians, is not encouraging. However, the very close family ties and mutual responsibilities which now make up such an essential part of the lives of Pakistani immigrants are likely to endure for at least two or three generations, providing both supports and frustrations for the families concerned. The social workers who help these families will need to be very much aware of the tightly knit social background which both prompted and sustained the Pakistani immigration, as well as the importance of religious and cultural traditions for people whose nationality and identity exist in their fantasy and imagination as well as in reality.

Indians in Britain

Indian immigrants in Britain come almost exclusively from two areas. The Sikhs, who make up approximately four-fifths of Indian immigrants, are from the Jullundur and Hoshiarpur districts of East Punjab where in some villages one in ten of the original inhabitants is in the UK. The second area of emigration is Gujarat, north of Bombay. Gujarati immigrants are mainly Hindus.

Indian immigrants are in many ways similar to those from Pakistan in that many of them are traditionally peasants who for various reasons have been unable to eke out a living on the land and so have migrated to industrial areas. In Britain they have settled mainly in the Midlands and London, where they have found work as unskilled labourers and in transport. Like the Pakistani immigrants, both Sikhs and Gujaratis have a tradition of migration which is, therefore, a natural solution to the poverty, frustration, and political upheaval they may experience in India and which also helps them to organize and sustain the complications of travel to and settlement in unfamiliar countries. Similarly, their migration is sponsored by relatives, and this leads, certainly in the early years, to the establishment of close links between families in India and their absent members in Britain.

The joint family system, common amongst many Indians —especially those of the peasant classes—not only involves all the rights and obligations of the extended family but can also mean that a family of different generations consisting of parents, their married sons with their wives and children, and their unmarried children will live in the same house. Money and possessions are held in common and the conduct of family affairs is a communal activity, although there is some privacy for husbands and wives. The drift of peasants from the land and the earning of individual wages, which are not so easily shared, are weakening the organization of the joint family; nevertheless, it still exercises an important influence in the lives of many Indians and can be even more binding than the rather looser network of the extended family. The joint family system does not exist only when there is shared accommodation. Its bonds and responsibilities continue when relatives are living apart. Certainly in Britain the kinship groups of Indian immigrants—and since these are large they will include, by implication, the village groups of their homelands—are the focus of their lives, providing them with material and emotional security. Within these kinship groups men still outnumber women, although the sexes are more evenly balanced than amongst Pakistani immigrants, since the Sikhs began to bring their wives and families to Britain as soon as immigration controls were anticipated. As with the Pakistanis, the establishment of their families meant an improvement in the standard of living of the original Indian migrants.

The Sikhs

The Sikhs are some of the most able and versatile people in India and have for centuries travelled abroad as pedlars or as skilled or semi-skilled employees working on large engineering projects. They have a long tradition of service in the Indian army, and their abilities and perseverance have led to their being sponsored as frontiersmen or pioneers in opening up under-developed regions of India. This has all been achieved in spite of a high level of illiteracy amongst Sikhs, whose main spoken language is Punjabi. They are able to converse with other Indians either through the medium of simple Hindi or English, which is spoken to some degree by about half of the male Sikh immigrants in Britain.

During their rule of India, the British felt more affinity with the Sikhs than they did with most of their Indian subjects, and admired their qualities and encouraged their loyalty. Amongst older Sikhs and English people, some remnants of this relationship still exist.

1 *Religious beliefs* Sikh religious beliefs and social organization lie at the root of their success. Their faith was founded in the sixteenth century by Guru Nanak and was developed and consolidated by the nine gurus, or teachers, who followed him during the next two hundred years. Essentially Sikhism developed as a protest against the excessive ritualism, idolatry, and social divisions which then characterized Hinduism; it sought also to incorporate both Hindu and Moslem traditions, and the Sikh holy book, the Granth Sahib, bears witness to this. Sikhs believe in the oneness of God and the equality of all men, thus denying the validity of the caste system. Orthodox Sikhs believe that they belong to a brotherhood, and the adoption of a common name, Singh (a lion) by men and Kaur

(a princess) by women, served to remove the caste distinction revealed in the family name. Some male Sikhs also observe certain customs of dress, of which the most obvious and familiar is the tradition of wearing the hair and beard unshorn. Orthodox Sikhs will also abstain from beef, tobacco, and, strictly speaking, alcohol. Although they have not been entirely successful in removing the influences of the caste system, Sikhs recognize a common identity and mutual obligations which work greatly to their advantage, particularly when they are in foreign countries. This recognition of common bonds and obligations has made possible some association between the Sikh landless peasants and the educated élite who, partly from force of circumstances, have taken on manual work which would be considered impossible by those who adhere to a strict caste system. These more educated Sikhs have also acted as intermediaries and leaders, and, as a result, Indian immigrant organizations, although often subject to internal disputes, have made some impact both on English society and amongst Indian immigrants themselves. In particular, most sizeable Sikh communities establish a gurudwara which, as both a temple and social centre, provides them with a focus and common meeting-place.

Some Sikhs believe that the orthodox practice of their religious traditions, apart from its intrinsic value, is an essential part of the maintenance of their special identity and mutual support. They emphasize the importance of the Sikhs as a religious, semi-national group. Others believe that the preservation of a separate identity, particularly by such outward symbols as the wearing of the turban, is not essential to the maintenance of Sikh values and may also be inimical to their settlement in foreign countries. Such issues can be highly controversial and emotional, and it is likely that Sikh families will contain, perhaps indefinitely, strictly orthodox and more liberal members. This will depend partly on the nature of the contacts Sikhs preserve with their original homelands and their religious traditions. Although we do not yet know the extent to which young Sikhs will be influenced by the social and religious traditions of their families, as well as the values implicit in their British education, it is likely that they will challenge strict orthodoxy, while possibly recognizing some traditional bonds amongst Sikhs.

A further important factor in Sikh religious tradition is the emphasis placed on the necessity for men to exercise some control over their destiny. Early persecution of the Sikhs forced them to become a militant organization, and the establishment and protection of their rights did not accord with submission to the Divine Will and the acceptance of fate, however unpleasant. The Sikh searches for God not by renouncing the world and its ways but through deep involvement with them. This view of the role of man and his destiny is familiar and sympathetic to those brought up in Western cultural traditions and provides a potential basis for some common understanding between Sikhs and Europeans.

2 *Family traditions* Although men are the undisputed heads of Sikh families, women exercise an important influence and are not nearly as restricted and confined as Moslem women. Their social life, including their contact with men, is much greater, and there is also some tradition of employment for women which contributes to greater equality between Sikh men and women. This greater equality between the sexes, combined with the fact that many men stay in their family of origin all their lives, can result in very close relationships between a mother and her sons to the exclusion of their wives. This relationship is further influenced by the long absence, through migration, of the fathers and heads of families, which can also leave the senior female family members, especially the grandmothers, in a powerful position. In spite of this more equal distribution of influence, the public relation-

ships between Sikh men and women, as in Moslem families, are formal and do not allow for open expression of feeling.

Although an important part of the social organization of Indians, the joint family system can be the source of friction as well as security, particularly for those women who recognize and accept some measure of independence and equality with men. Sikh women who migrate to Britain and find this family structure much modified, while missing its companionship, may appreciate the greater degree of freedom it allows. Unlike Moslem women, it is possible for them to find some satisfaction outside the immediate domesticity of the family, even through employment outside the home. However, although Indians may recognize substantial differences in their family organization, to English people its relationships will appear very close knit, extended, and quite unlike the two-generation households which are most common in Britain.

Sikh children, especially during their adolesence, are strictly brought up to recognize their obligations to family members and to the wider Sikh community. There is, however, less emphasis on the isolation and protection of girls and on the superiority of boys than in Moslem families, and although parents arrange the marriages of their children, they are usually allowed to express some opinion about the choice made and even to veto it. However, Sikh parents in Britain are likely, certainly for the next decade or so, to try to maintain village and kinship solidarity, including giving some consideration to caste obligations through the marriage of their children.

Indians from Gujarat

Gujarati Indians also have a long tradition of migration and, in particular, many have settled in East Africa, where they have established substantial commercial interests and are recognized as a highly successful middle-class group. The political upheavals in Africa are forcing many of these expatriate Indians to migrate once again, and those who do manage to enter Britain, in spite of the severe restrictions on their immigration, represent some of the more cosmopolitan, able, and adaptable immigrants. Those immigrants who come straight from Gujarat have not had such extensive contact with Western cultural influences, although many of them have some experience of urban life and most are literate. The most commonly used language is Gujarati.

1 *Hindu religious and social traditions* Most Gujarati immigrants are, or have been, members of joint families, and the great majority are Hindus, although they have adapted some of the religious tenets and social practices of Hinduism in the course of their migration. Hinduism is one of the oldest religions in the world and by far the most common in India. Its beliefs are complex, but at their basis they involve the worship of a number of gods and goddesses of whom the most important are Brahma, the Creator, Vishnu, the Preserver, and Shiva, the Destroyer. Hinduism is a sacramental religion, and its festivals, which are rich in ceremonial, provide an important social and emotional focus for many Indians. Hindus also believe in the transmigration of souls, and accept that all living beings are the same in essence. Traditional Hinduism also upholds the division of society into fixed social classes or castes. Hindus are forbidden to eat beef and most are vegetarians.

The caste system is very complicated; although four main classes are recognized, there is a multiplicity of sub-castes. Originally, the caste system, based on occupational groups and so promoting the organized division of labour, was intended to provide an orderly and peaceful society. However, in its strict interpretation it prevented any social mobility and encouraged divisions within society, whereby the members of lower castes were severely repressed by those of higher castes. Traditionally, contact between members of different castes, ranging from marriage to eating together, and even to touching each other, involved pollution and was forbidden. Castes also provide strict codes of conduct, and any deviation from these and other obligations of caste means cutting oneself off from the family and kinship group and the security and protection these provide. Since migration inevitably involves some such contact, many Hindus would not think of undertaking it.

However, the caste system, while still influential in India, particularly in social life, has been severely modified. Not only does it have no legal sanction, but the requirements of urban living, complicated industrialization, and the acquisition of individual wealth, despite caste membership, make it impossible for caste to survive in its strict form. Indians who migrate are those who are more willing and able to adapt or modify the obligations of the caste system or those who are anxious to escape from its restraints. Immigrant Indians are afforded high status within their own communities not because of their caste but according to their practical achievements, such as their ability to speak English and their ownership of property. None the less, partly because of their close links with their native village communities, where at least the social obligations of caste still hold sway, many Indian immigrants are influenced in their choice of marriage partners, and sometimes their business associates, by considerations of caste. Some observers also believe that these traditions are so strong and deep rooted that fears of breaking caste rules and obligations linger, although perhaps barely consciously, even amongst some apparently very liberal Indians. Such anxieties could influence even their closest relationships.

2 *Family life* In orthodox Hindu families, a woman's place is an essentially humble one, and particularly when she is first married, an Indian girl is expected to sub-

ordinate all her wishes to those of her husband's family, particularly her mother-in-law. It is considered both her duty and her desire to please and serve her husband for whom she will bear a special reverence. Depending on the welcome she finds in her new family, marriage may, therefore, be a traumatic event. Although in India divorce is possible, most Hindus regard marriages as indissoluble and do not even expect widows to remarry. Even more than with the Sikhs, the bond between mother and son is strong, as is the relationship between brother and sister. Like Moslems and Sikhs, Hindu children are brought up to recognize their obligations to the joint family system, and from early childhood girls are prepared to accept their devoted but humble position as wives.

Amongst Gujarati Indians, men still significantly out-number women and it is not easy to predict how reunited Hindu families will adapt to life in Britain. What is clear, however, is that those Hindus who migrate are amongst the more liberal and flexible and so are unlikely to abide rigidly by religious traditions and the social obligations these involve. This flexibility could be further influenced by the fact that Hindu religious observance in foreign countries is centred on the home and there is no provision for organized worship outside this context. However, the family and village group will remain of supreme impor-tance to the Gujarati Indians in Britain. Desai (1963) has described the web of mutual support and obligations that surrounds their lives, assuring them of accommodation, employment, leisure activities, and contact with their families in India. Indian commercial enterprises provide their practical necessities, and various associations seek to promote their interests as a national group. These are 'the social walls which both imprison and protect them' (p. 121).

Indians and migration

In what way and for how long these walls will survive is
not clear. Both Sikhs and Gujaratis have proved themselves
most capable immigrants to countries other than Britain,
and there is some evidence that they have maintained over
long periods some national, cultural, and religious identity.
Unlike Moslems, who may marry Christians and Jews,
Sikhs and Hindus are not permitted to marry members of
different faiths, and to do so may mean rejection by the
rest of the family. Social contact with English women is
not, therefore, likely to be welcomed. Although there can
be serious disputes within Gujarati and Sikh communities,
these are most usually settled internally; Indians are
anxious not to bring themselves into disrepute by seeking
help with these and other difficulties. Their relatively
secure and united families and their own cultural traditions also make it unlikely that they will seek the help of
the social services with domestic problems. Nevertheless,
the contraction of the family unit, which is an inevitable
consequence of migration, will eventually mean that
Indians are more dependent on the agencies of the state.
It is also possible that Indian child-rearing practices—
which are in many ways the opposite of those common in
England in that Indians tend to indulge young children but
treat adolescents strictly—may be the source of some
friction amongst those families whose children have grown
up within the English educational system.

Those social workers who have had contact with Indian
families, while feeling very much that they are seen as
outsiders and representatives of a culture that is in many
ways alien, find that relationships are more easily established than with Pakistani families. This may partly arise
because Hindu and Sikh philosophy, while being very strict
in some respects, can also encourage a breadth of vision
and some tolerance for alternative patterns of life. The
Indian family described in Sharma's book (1971) illustrate

169

these qualities well. Easier relationships may also develop because a well-organized migration, such as that of the Indians, finds mutually acceptable ways of communicating with the native community. These relationships may also reflect the familiarity some Indians feel with the British as a result of their contact with them during Imperial rule. None the less, relations with officials are often characterized by a formal politeness which seems to indicate both a will to please and to hold outsiders at arm's length, frequently denying the need for any help external to the family. In the eyes of Europeans, relationships within the Indian family itself can appear formal and somewhat inhibited.

During the next few years, social workers are most likely to have contact with those Indian immigrants who, for various reasons, find themselves outcasts of their own community. These may be people who have seriously offended against religious or social mores, or possibly better educated Indians who feel that there is little satisfaction for them in India or amongst the immigrant community, and yet who are unable to find a place in English society that fits their abilities and aspirations. These are the Indians most likely to form relationships with English people; and while some of these will be most successful and mutually satisfying, others may founder, both because of the differing expectations of the English and Indians and because of the social disapproval and rejection of such couples by both immigrants and natives. It is also possible that in the next decade or so social workers will meet disappointed and frustrated young Indians who will look for a place in British society, unlike their parents who expect to some extent to be discriminated against by the English. They may also emerge as a 'cultureless' group who feel they owe allegiance to neither Indian nor English traditions and who, therefore, feel rootless and isolated.

Conclusion

The policies and practices of the British government and people during the next ten to fifteen years will be critical in deciding the place of immigrants in English society. During this period, the extent of the influence of extended families, with their various cultural traditions, will also become clearer, but as Aurora (1968, p. 131) observes, at least during the early years of migration:

> cultural self sufficiency or the lack of it to some extent guides the behaviour of communities towards the host society. Since the Indo-Pakistanis cherish their separate identity and stand guard against the 'pernicious' influences of the host society, they expect less intimacy and consideration from it; while the West Indian, being oriented differently, expects much greater consideration and in his heart passionately desires greater intimacy which through bitter experience he learns to be frustrated.

This accounts for some of the aggression many West Indians feel towards English society and their increasing wish to withdraw and form their own organizations in an attempt to achieve the kind of protection and support experienced by immigrants from India and Pakistan.

6

Social work methods and policy

> Anything that obscures the fundamentally moral nature of the social problem is harmful, no matter whether it proceeds from the side of physical or psychological theory. Any doctrine that eliminates or even obscures the function of choice of values and enlistment of desires and emotions in belief of those chosen weakens personal responsibility for judgement and for action (Dewey, 1940, p. 172).

Previous chapters have shown how much overlap there is between the problems of immigrants and those of other minority groups, especially those living in the poorest urban areas, and how their presence highlights the short-comings and anomalies of the social services, including the activities of social workers. Those social policies which alleviate the problems of immigrants will, therefore, meet the needs of many of the indigenous population.

There are also some special features in the background and settlement of immigrants in Britain which distinguish them from most natives and which will influence the demands they make on the social services and their response to them. Social workers sometimes find that their contact with immigrants raises fundamental questions of social work policy and technique; by throwing into relief assumptions underlying approaches to the solving of problems, immigrants act as a catalyst in more general thinking about the functions and methods of social work.

This chapter can only mention briefly those social work issues which are spotlighted by the demands of

172

immigrants but which concern many of those who need social work help. The final section of this volume has a guide to further reading about these subjects. In this chapter, rather more time will be spent discussing aspects of social work policy and technique which are especially relevant in helping immigrants and their families.

Some general issues

Chapter 3 has shown how discussion about meeting the needs of the most deprived members of society, amongst whom are numbered many immigrants, must be a discussion about politics and social policy more than about social work. None the less, social work has a part to play in the alleviation of the problems of the underprivileged, and the demands made on the profession and the observations of its many critics are leading to a reassessment of its role.

1 *The limitations of social work* In the first place, the limitations of social work are now being more openly acknowledged. Perlman (1969), Plowman (1969), and Holman and Radford (1969), to mention only a few, have suggested that casework is an effective, appropriate method helping only in certain defined circumstances which include an adequate economic and material environment. Marris and Rein (1967), Halsey (1971), and Holman (1970), amongst many others, have discussed the function and limitations of community work programmes and have emphasized the importance of the political context in which they operate. Social work may alleviate but cannot remove the gross inequalities in society and the suffering these entail. Nevertheless, as several of the case studies have illustrated, social work has a very real contribution to make in helping individuals and families who are burdened with serious personal and environmental problems.

2 *Control over material resources* Increasing awareness

of the poverty of many of those who need social work help has resulted in social workers being given more control over material resources, although Sinfield (1969) and other critics argue that this is still far too restricted, partly because social workers have not pressed for even greater control. These critics also point to the way in which clients' access to certain resources is limited or prevented by the failure of social work agencies to inform them of their rights and to explain the existence and function of social services and legal and administrative machinery. Chapter 3 has shown how these questions of the allocation of social resources, and of access to social services, are especially relevant to those areas in which most immigrants live.

3 *Long- or short-term help* Social workers and administrators have in recent years been much concerned about the most effective focus of social work services. Some emphasis is now placed on providing help for families and individuals whose problems are at an early stage of development, to prevent deterioration into crisis or chronic difficulty. Sometimes help is also made available to those whose particular circumstances make it likely that they will be receptive to some special and usually short-term help, which, if given, will contribute substantially to the future well-being of the individuals concerned. The focus of this help is on the normal 'crises' in the life cycle of most individuals. These assumptions underlie the provision of special services for mothers and young children, the recently bereaved, or those about to retire. However, the scope and range of preventive services are likely to be limited, not only because of the relatively restricted resources available to them, but also because they raise complex questions of social philosophy concerning the extent of the responsibility of the state to intervene in family life, and of the individual to fend for himself. For example, although it can be argued that the many prob-

lems surrounding migration call for some special help for immigrants, there is also anxiety that the provision of help might impose unjustified pressure to conform and adapt to a way of life deemed appropriate by social workers and administrators, but unacceptable to immigrants and their families. Chapter 1 described the understandable resistance to singling out immigrants for special attention and, to a large extent, it is thought both right and proper that they should make their own way in their new country. The problems and suffering this will mean for them and the implications of these for the provision of some special help are usually ignored.

Another expression of this concern with the focus and content of services can be seen in the current preoccupation of social workers with the different merits of giving long-term support or short-term intensive help. The problems of immigrants provide a useful context in which these questions can be clarified. For example, Anthea and her parents might have escaped some suffering if they had received some intensive help immediately after their reunion, whereas the Khan family needed prolonged contact with a social worker while they grappled with their problems.

4 *The power and influence of social workers* Social workers are currently very aware that much of their work involves influencing individuals or groups to behave in certain ways. This influence can reflect the humanitarian values of social work as, for instance, when social workers try to prevail on organizations or individuals to provide resources and to show consideration for particularly needy but not widely accepted people, such as unmarried mothers and their children. But the influence of social workers can also reflect some of the dominant values of society; this is illustrated, for example, in the pressures social workers put on people to find and stay in employment, or to provide for themselves wherever possible, sometimes even to the extent of ignoring difficulties which individuals cannot

satisfactorily solve on their own.

In their contact with immigrants, especially if they are coloured, social workers will be much influenced by their own personal views and the prevailing attitudes of society. Chapter 1 discussed some of the different perceptions of immigrants; and social workers, like many others, will be uncertain both about which is the most appropriate and helpful, and about the consequent implications for social policy. The varying backgrounds and needs of different immigrant groups make some of this confusion unavoidable, and social workers will find that some of their activities imply that immigrants want or ought to adapt or assimilate to British society, while others take account of their wish to maintain distinctive cultural traditions. In understanding the conflict which inevitably accompanies the settlement of immigrants, social workers need to be clear about the ways in which their own influence contributes to this and how this influence is shaped by personal and professional values. The probation officer in the Williamson case was caught in this dilemma.

5 *The participation of clients* Very much connected with this awareness of the influence of social workers is the increasing recognition that the people who use the social services should have more influence in determining their policies. Although most social workers accept this in principle, they are naturally ambivalent about the criticism of their activities which this participation can involve and anxious about the pressures which may be brought on them to adapt their policies and methods. The wishes and demands of organizations concerned with immigrants, and the reaction of social workers, provide useful illustrations of the complexities of co-operation between the users and the providers of the social services.

6 *The selectivity of the social services* Finally, in their use of the social services, immigrants spotlight fundamental

questions about the universality of these services and the discretionary powers of officials to allocate those resources which are intended only to meet exceptional needs. For example, there is some relief that the immigrants' over-all age structure means that they contribute, through taxes and other means, more to the social services than they take out; we are gratified that they make full and appropriate use of most 'universal' services concerned with health and education. But social workers can also be irritated by some immigrants' failure to distinguish between the aims and functions of other social services. They do not always appreciate that a sophisticated understanding of social services, and long familiarity with them, is needed before distinctions can be made between those services which are considered to be everyone's right and those to which people are only expected to turn as a last resort. And since ideas about the universality of provision are always in a state of flux, these distinctions can never be absolutely clear; a person's eligibility for many services may depend on the availability of resources and an official's estimation of his need rather than on any agreed criteria. The demands of immigrants draw attention to the ways social workers reach such decisions. Their response to requests for children to be cared for outside their own homes vividly illustrates this confusion in balancing needs and rights.

Some special needs of immigrants

Given these general preoccupations and concerns of social work, underlined by the needs of immigrants and of importance to them, what special awareness should there be of their particular problems?

1   *Pre-school children*   The isolation of many immigrant families and the material hardship they experience, place their pre-school children in an especially vulnerable posi-

tion. Young West Indian children are perhaps the most at risk. The previous chapter described the strains on their families which contribute to this vulnerability and their special need for adequate daily care in the absence of their working mothers. Although usually more protected and supported by their family network, young Asian children and their mothers may be helped to establish contact with the outside world by attendance at playgroups, which eases the sometimes traumatic transition from home to school. Serious difficulties may also face those families whose children are privately fostered while their parents are at work or studying and whose sole purpose in coming to Britain may have been to obtain a qualification.

The policy of most departments not to receive into care the children of married couples who are both at work, while understandable in many ways, forces these parents into the dubious arena of the private minder; and frequently they, or the foster-parents they find, are blamed for providing inadequate child care. There are direct parallels here with those housing authorities, unable or unwilling to provide accommodation for newcomers, which prosecute the landlords who do meet these needs, albeit in unsatisfactory ways. If departments feel obliged not to provide care for children whose parents insist that temporarily they are unable to care for them themselves, they must at least do all in their power to ensure that alternative arrangements are satisfactory and, where necessary, take steps to improve them by providing help for foster-parents, and perhaps, some special services, such as extra play facilities, for their charges. The extension of Child Protection legislation goes some way to meeting these problems, but there is evidence that the supervision of private foster homes is variable, sometimes consisting only of infrequent official oversight with little help being offered either to the foster-parents, their foster-children, or the natural parents.

2 *Relationships between parents and adolescents* It is likely that some immigrant families who settle in Britain will face difficult problems of relationship with their adolescent children. Although most families will cope with these difficulties without serious disruption, some organizations, including schools and youth clubs, believe that it is helpful to offer counselling services or group support for the parents and children in this predicament. Some immigrants may prefer these services to be conducted under the auspices of their own organizations and to be designed especially for their particular national groups. Although they may have problems similar to those of parents of different cultural backgrounds, careful consideration needs to be given to preferences to meet in familiar circumstances which give some security. Eisenstadt (1954) has shown that those immigrants who settled most easily in Israel belonged to cohesive family units which maintained, initially at least, a lively awareness of their national identity. There are grave risks in insisting for doctrinaire reasons that, at a relatively early stage of their settlement, people should share all their activities with those whose values and cultures may be quite unfamiliar and unsympathetic. These issues have been more fully discussed in the Hunt Report on *Immigrants and the Youth Service* (1967). Groups for isolated Indian or Pakistani women, perhaps focused on activities or English language classes in their own homes, may also be useful.

3 *Practical help and advice* Partly because of their unfamiliarity with immigrants, social workers are sometimes inclined to exaggerate the serious and chronic nature of their problems. There will of course be those who had serious problems before their migration which will continue, and perhaps be aggravated, in their new country. There will also be some families whose migration lies at the root of their problems in that it has involved damaging separations. The case of Anthea is one example. Other

immigrants may face such chronic problems of housing, education, and employment that it becomes impossible for them to establish themselves satisfactorily and happily in Britain. However, most commonly, immigrants will experience difficulties—very often arising directly from their migration—which, although acute, will be temporary. Some of these problems are described in chapter 4.

Such crises call initially for intensive but short-term work with a special focus on practical help and encouragement. In cases where social workers suspect that the crisis of migration has reactivated an individual's earlier problems, at times when he is faced with severe practical difficulties and in a lonely and dependent state, the immigrant client is unlikely to be able to connect past and present experiences, nor would it be helpful at this stage for him to do so. Assessment of the long-term incapacity and need for prolonged assistance can only be made realistically after short-term and intensive help has been offered. Frequently the help needed will include advice and explanation about the function of the various social services and the legal rights of immigrants. When their most immediate anxieties are focused on the problems of bringing relatives to Britain and they are caught up in a tangle of regulations and bureaucracy, which do not always work in their favour, immigrants may need expert help with these difficulties. However, since few people are anxious to assist the entry of more immigrants in to Britain, whatever may be their rights, this help is frequently not forthcoming. The resulting family distress can be acute. Most social workers will not have the necessary detailed information about immigration regulations, and they should, therefore, help immigrants to contact the local community relations council, the UK Immigrants' Advisory Service, or the Joint Council for the Welfare of Immigrants. Details of these organizations are given at the end of the final section of this volume.

The contribution of casework

A lively awareness of the limitations of the various methods of social work should not prevent us from acknowledging and defining its role in meeting human needs. When discussing the circumstances of the under-privileged, there is sometimes an unfair tendency to assume that caseworkers, more than most other social workers, will have little to contribute to the solution of their problems. This assumption frequently arises from a misunder-standing of the function and methods of casework. Equally, in focusing on the very real material needs of de-prived people, this view can often disregard their personal problems of family relationships, loneliness, discontent-ment, and anxiety.

These problems may well arise from the general poverty which encircles the lives of many social work clients. Case-workers must and can involve themselves with this outer world of their clients and work for its improvement. That they are able to do this in significant ways is illustrated by the activities of the groups of social workers described in chapter 3. Nevertheless, deep-rooted misunderstandings and bitterness between relatives and some of the con-sequences of the inevitable neglect of children who live in a poor environment, will not simply disappear as a family's material circumstances improve, even if this can be achieved. In these cases, caseworkers may have to help their clients to explore the inner world of feelings and emotions and, perhaps, to give vent to pent-up tensions. They may also need to help people to understand, tolerate, or endure the behaviour of their relatives, which gives rise to so much pain. One of the main strengths of casework is its focus on individual need, and we should not imagine that attempting to ease the personal suffering of individuals means condoning the circumstances which contribute to it. Like all other social workers, caseworkers have a role to play in a wider and more political context.

As several of the case studies have illustrated, there will be many immigrants whose problems are concerned with the disruption of family relationships and the almost inevitable changes in role, aspiration, and outlook which accompany migration. The immigrants' shock and bewilderment at their completely new environment may need sensitive understanding and cushioning. These problems were described in chapter 4. Caseworkers can have a major role to play in helping immigrants and their families understand, and so tolerate better, their reactions to their changing world. As the case studies of the Khan and Williamson families show, caseworkers can also help immigrants to have the confidence to take the risk of experimenting with new roles and ideas. Within this relationship too it is possible to weigh up the losses and gains of migration without fear of criticism or recrimination.

Some aspects of casework with immigrants

Although some of the problems discussed in the next section have a bearing on all social work methods, they are particularly relevant to casework.

1 *Communication between immigrants and social workers* Too great an emphasis on problems of communication can sometimes form a barrier behind which immigrants and natives hide, with much stress being placed on the importance of understanding each other's traditions as a necessary stepping-stone to communication. The two cannot be separated. Attempts to study the values and customs of groups with whom there is no contact can serve only to highlight strange differences between them which, taken out of context, are often grossly misunderstood. In other contexts, social workers are very familiar with the two-way process whereby, as they begin to make a relationship with a family, its history and aspirations unfold; equally, this growing understanding is accompanied by a stronger

relationship between them and the family concerned.

Apart from problems of communication arising from straightforward language difficulties involving the use of interpreters, different conceptions of the importance of punctuality also contribute to misunderstandings. Attention paid to timekeeping is a mark of industrial societies and may be quite unfamiliar to many immigrants who find it hard, in the early stages of their contact with social work agencies, to comprehend the importance of making and keeping appointments. They may also see a social worker's tendency to fix special times for visits to families as excessively formal. Failure to keep appointments should, therefore, not necessarily be interpreted as an immigrant's unwillingness to receive help, although when an initial contact has been established, social workers may need to discuss with their immigrant clients plans for keeping in touch with each other.

Complications may also arise when immigrants ask for help at a very late stage in their difficulties, either because of their prolonged efforts to solve them themselves, or because they have been misinformed about where to seek appropriate help. Social workers may be angry that they have been consulted so late and immigrants resentful of their delays in giving help while enquiries are being made.

Possibly because of this delay in obtaining appropriate help, or because many immigrants are unused to discussing their difficulties and unsure about the response of social workers or the kind of help available, some problems tend to be presented in a most dramatic way. There can be vivid accounts of violently disobedient children, wife-beating husbands, promiscuous wives, and demands that one or other party should be removed or controlled. While these stories may be substantially true, they can also reflect the ways in which some family members, immigrant and native, unused to discussion and very much under stress, communicate with each other and with the outside world. It does not necessarily mean that there are no alternatives to the separation of the feuding parties. Nevertheless, there is a real danger that social workers, faced with situations which seem unfamiliar more because of the background of the individuals contributing to them than their actual nature, may panic and take drastic and sometimes premature action. There is always some risk in failing to respond to apparently urgent problems in the ways demanded by the people who present them, but with immigrants—as much as, and perhaps more than, with other clients—social workers need to try to acquaint themselves as fully as possible with the nature of the relationships between different family members and the background to the present crisis and request for help. The case study of the Williamson family illustrates many of these difficulties.

Like many people who are unused to discussing personal or family problems, immigrants sometimes complain initially of physical symptoms which seem to have little organic basis. If they admit to being depressed, they will, on occasions, explain this by accounts of the ways they are being persecuted by neighbours or relatives, or they may simply say they have been cursed by God. Social workers may see such complaints as indications of psychiatric illness. However, in a review of the numerous studies of psychiatric illness amongst immigrants, Bagley (1968) emphasizes the importance of understanding apparently psychiatric symptoms in the context of the general stresses of immigration. Seemingly paranoid ideas often have their root in the discrimination and prejudice most immigrants encounter in their everyday lives; they are sometimes unwilling to acknowledge these and so project their rejection onto those nearest them. A belief in the disfavour of the Deity has to be understood in terms of teachings and traditions which emphasize the arbitrariness of Fate and the need to submit to it. Such beliefs flourish in countries where little has been done to protect their inhabitants from the cruellest influences of the environment. Overall, the incidence of psychiatric illness amongst immigrants is not thought to vary very significantly from that of the general population.

Even when not under stress, different nationalities have characteristic ways of expressing themselves. West Indians and Cypriots are generally more voluble and emotional than Indians and Pakistanis, who pride themselves on control of their feelings. They may, therefore, be mystified and upset by the apparent reserve and chilliness of British people, who frequently recoil when faced with behaviour they regard as uncontrolled. Not surprisingly, many immigrants do not know how they are received by British people nor what is expected of them. There can be added complications when, for reasons described in previous chapters, immigrants see people in authority in the context of colonial experience and traditions. Social workers may, therefore, need to make more explicit to their immigrant clients their views, their approval and disapproval, their warmth and concern, if they are not to add to the confusion immigrants already feel.

It is not always easy for social workers to adapt the kind of responses they make to their clients, particularly if they feel ill at ease with them. Some of this discomfort arises from their unfamiliarity with immigrants which will disappear with more frequent contact. It can also be associated with the resentment, sometimes barely conscious, that social workers feel when confronted with the demands, and even the presence, of coloured immigrants. This resentment and anger may arise from misunderstandings, or it may be connected with the threat immigrants are seen to present to cherished ideals such as those concerned with child care, marital relationships, or individual responsibility. In those circles most conscious of the injustice and discrimination against immigrants, and anxious to display their own impartiality, it can be difficult for such feelings to be discussed openly and helpfully. Senior workers have a responsibility to help their colleagues air these issues in general terms and in connection with particular cases. There is no advantage to be gained in ignoring feelings and attitudes which, if suppressed, make social work ineffective or more difficult.

2 *Relationships between immigrants and social workers*
(a) Authority and dependence. Possibly because establishing communication sometimes calls for special efforts on the part of immigrants and social workers, the relationships between them can be characterized by an unusual degree of warmth and vitality. However, some social workers are surprised and rather alarmed by the apparent dependence of their immigrant clients on them. They are reluctant to play the roles of adviser and arbitrator, and recoil from taking the kind of direct and immediate action which immigrants sometimes demand of them. To behave in this way seems contrary to the important principle that people who come for social work help should as far as possible direct their own affairs and make their own decisions.

They may also recoil from these roles because of their subtle attraction. A relationship which depends on one person being seen as the 'expert master' and the other as the dependent and grateful client is a seductive one which haunted social work earlier in this century and of which we are now rightly wary. Nevertheless, in their anxiety to avoid this trap, some social workers fail to recognize or meet their immigrant clients' dependency needs which may be acute, although usually short-lived. Previous chapters have shown how this dependence may be connected with the regression many people experience when faced with the stresses of immigration, how it may be influenced by immigrants' views of the role of social workers and occasionally by their belief, generally transistory, that they have no control over their destiny. The father of the family in Sharma's book (1971, p. 23) speaks for many immigrants when he says: 'Every child that is born has its own apportioned fate; some are born into ease and joy, others into trouble and suffering... we cannot say why these things happen, only that they do happen ...'. Such a religious and philosophical outlook, born of necessary resignation to centuries of overwhelming suffering, is nevertheless countered by the obvious eagerness of immigrants to mould their own futures. Understood in this context, the immigrants' temporary dependence and passivity need not make social workers unduly anxious when they are asked to play more positive roles than they would expect with many of their native clients. In most cases this is a necessary step towards helping individuals re-establish the independence and abilities which made their migration possible and which will help them undertake the enterprises and endure the hardships which are an essential part of settlement in a new country.

Such a relationship may involve a social worker in giving very practical help, advice, or explanation concerning housing, employment, and the care of children. This can include accompanying people to unfamiliar agencies, making their problems known, and negotiating on their behalf. However, some of the problems of immigrants will be more complex and may involve a considerable degree of conflict both within families, between immigrants, and between immigrants and natives. In these situations social workers often feel it is inappropriate to give advice, although they may need to be quite explicit about the different lines of action which could be adopted, where possible indicating their likely outcome. Social workers also have to make it clear why they are unable to give direct advice, explaining that responsibility for decisions must rest with the immigrant family or individual. Like many other people, some immigrants try to avoid involving themselves in too much personal responsibility; they are frightened of being branded as failures both by their own relatives and by the community which tolerates them only on sufferance. Social workers may be amongst the few people who can show immigrants that it is possible to fail and yet not be rejected, supporting them in taking the risks involved in establishing independence and helping them to tolerate better the failures of others, especially their children.

(b) Insight and reflection. This emphasis on practical help, advice and direction, encouragement and support does not mean that there are not many occasions when it is helpful to explore with immigrants the emotional background to some of their problems, but care should be taken in assessing when this is appropriate. Faced with the numerous practical difficulties of migration, thinking about oneself and one's relationships can seem an unnecessary luxury. Some immigrants, too, may need to defend themselves against their acute loneliness and sense of loss by heavy involvement in various activities, and it is not always helpful to distract them from this. When immigrants do discuss their own feelings and family relationships, social workers need more than ever to listen rather than offer their own interpretations and comments, so that they can form a meaningful picture of a network of commitments, expectations, and relationships which are unfamiliar to most Europeans. This was the role successfully adopted by the social worker concerned with the Khan family.

(d) Personal responses. The warmth, acceptance, and support that social workers are able to offer immigrants must be the foundation of their work with them. Since most immigrants have little conception of a professional social work relationship, once they feel at ease, their response is not inhibited by the constraints that some people believe are its necessary or inevitable accompaniments, and their approach may be personal and social. They may want to know something of the private lives of their social workers and often respond in a lively way to accounts of their families. They sometimes give small presents and offer hospitality, occasionally inviting social workers to parties or other celebrations. These attempts to establish a social worker as a real person can mean that he is no longer seen as a remote individual to whom deference must be paid. He may be the only white person with whom an immigrant client has any kind of personal contact, and it would be a pity if a somewhat rigid conception of a professional relationship limited this in unnecessary ways.

(e) Colour. 'Yes, it does indeed mean something—something unspeakable—to be born in a white country, an Anglo-Teutonic, anti-sexual country, black' (Baldwin, 1970, p. 33).

In their relationships with immigrants, whether these seem to be warm or distant, social workers need to realize that many coloured people will view them with deep suspicion as potential sources of rebuff and discrimination. These suspicions reflect the age-long exploitation of the black races by the white, and although they may decrease as relationships become well established, they may never completely disappear. Frequently these feelings are not openly expressed, although there are often many signs that coloured people think they are receiving an inferior service. Because social workers are annoyed by accusations they regard as untrue, or uneasy if they believe there is some substance to them, they usually avoid discussing these questions. In most cases this is unhelpful, since it leaves social workers and their coloured clients uncomfortable and resentful. Doubts and suspicions will not necessarily disappear if they are voiced, but if they are not recognized there is a greater chance of their festering and forming an obstacle of unknown proportions.

This unease and embarrassment is also reflected in some of the relationships between residential and field-workers and foster-parents and the coloured children in their care. Discussions about colour and its implications are usually avoided, and children are given no helpful explanations as to why they look different from their peers. The adults who care for them sometimes say that, at least while the children are young, they are themselves so unaware of these differences that it never seems appropriate to discuss them. This assertion is often belied by their openly expressed anxiety that, as the children grow older, it will be hard for them to gain acceptance in the wider community. It seems that the question of colour is so fraught with pain and fear that any opportunity to ignore it is seized. In the realms of fantasy these emotions assume even greater proportions.

(f) Failure and suffering. A few of the case studies quoted in an earlier chapter show that the process of migration has left deep and painful scars in the lives of some individuals. Anthea and Carol Ann's families were caught up in a process over which they could have little control. Equally, there will be some families who are overwhelmed by a constant battle with a hostile environment. Swallowed up in a bleak existence, with no hope of escape, they will see themselves as failures, objects of shame and ridicule to their relatives. These are people who may feel their lives and their struggle to have been in vain.

Social workers cannot remove this suffering. Nevertheless, we should not underestimate the value of relationships in which individuals feel warmly accepted for themselves rather than for their achievements. And since it is easier to ignore rather than acknowledge pain, so that many of those who endure it are left quite isolated, we should not forget that the open recognition of a person's grief can be helpful. Social workers are naturally affected by the suffering they witness, and in small but significant ways they share in this. There will be some immigrants who feel that the source and depth of their pain are known only to their social workers; and it is their social workers alone who have stayed with them in this. The value and strength of some human relationships lie in this quality of shared suffering.

3 *The conflict of cultures* 'The helping process must assume a certain quality of acculturation in which the worker tries to help the client move, at least somewhat, in the direction of the mental health culture which the family service and child welfare field in our society represent' (O. Pollak, 1965, p. 138).

Probably the most difficult dilemmas facing social workers are those which involve some conflict between the values and customs of immigrants and those of the society in which they have come to live. In both cases these traditions can be difficult to identify, and there are as many variations in the expectations of immigrants of different national groups as there are amongst British people. Most people do not expect immigrants to conform absolutely to the customs of their adopted country, and there is some respect for different cultural traditions. These attitudes hold, given some geographical and social distance between immigrants and natives. However, as O. Pollak (1962, p. 86) writes: 'When closeness is established, the proposition that one way of living may be as successful as another encounters a good deal of resistance'. There are also some risks in adopting an approach which assumes that immigrants should behave at all times according to their own customs, just because they are foreign and newcomers. This can lead to their being regarded with resentment as a deviant but privileged group; alternatively, they may be seen as inferior, rather in the way that slaves were, and unlikely to achieve any kind of equality with the dominant culture. As Rose (1969, p. 342) has argued; 'respect for other cultures can produce a pluralist solution based on parity of esteem; or it can tip over into "separate but equal"'.

It seems more appropriate, therefore, to expect immigrants to abide as far as possible by those customs and standards of behaviour which are regarded as essential in their new country. Identifying these requires some honesty, especially since the presence of immigrants can emphasize the weakness of our social structure and the shortcomings of our social policies and legislation. For example, many people recognize as cumbersome and inappropriate the legal procedures whereby unsupported mothers can claim financial support from the fathers of their children. Traditionally, West Indian women are most reluctant to adopt these measures. Should they therefore be pressed to do something which many people regard as unsatisfactory? Our social policies and legislation set great store on families providing for themselves wherever possible. Should we therefore encourage members of Asian families to seek help and alternative support outside this context? On the other hand, there are some standards of child care, some educational principles, and some beliefs about the position of women which we value highly, and we would see their abandonment as a most unfortunate return to the traditions of an earlier age which entailed acute suffering amongst some individuals. And yet many immigrants do not accept these principles and, indeed, may regard them as mistaken and dangerous. Social workers, magistrates, and teachers who are involved in the ensuing conflict are faced with deciding how far behaviour should be tolerated which is generally regarded as deviant by the majority, but which arises from sincerely held beliefs.

There is no easy answer to this question, and decisions must take into account the actual and likely suffering of the individuals concerned. However, in the anxiety to avoid such confrontations, two things are usually forgotten. In the first place, it is often too easily assumed that immigrants find their values and traditions challenged only in Britain. Many of those from rural backgrounds will already have found their conservatism seriously threatened in their native countries by the effects of ever-increasing industrialization and the widening of social legislation which usually accompanies this. Pressures on them to change some of their customs and adopt new ones are not, therefore, in themselves unfamiliar, although the extent of these pressures may be surprising.

Second and paradoxically, to be asked to conform to certain customs may indicate acceptance and a recognition of equality. This paradox is well illustrated by a conversation between a West Indian mother and a probation officer who was patiently trying to persuade her to adopt a more liberal attitude towards her teen-age daughter. The probation officer felt that the girl was only behaving in a way which was quite normal for her English friends, although her mother was adamant in her demands for total obedience, emphasizing that in their homeland such insolence and rebellion would not be tolerated. Suddenly the probation officer lost her temper, saying sharply: 'Well, your daughter is an English girl now, and you must accept that she will behave like other English girls'. Rather unexpectedly, and perhaps only because a basically good relationship existed between them, the mother smiled broadly, asking excitedly: 'Do you really think she can be English?' In situations which engender much criticism and bad feeling it is easy to forget that implicitly many immigrants recognize that their migration will involve some changes in their traditional way of life, and welcome the greater degree of acceptance that will ensue from these. Very few people are content to remain an isolated and alien minority. In the interests of everyone, the principle of cultural relativity, while initially appearing an attractive solution to conflict between immigrants and natives, needs careful examination.

Nevertheless, given these wishes and expectations of some adaptation, a substantial measure of personal and social security is needed before individuals are able to countenance changes in their own behaviour and that of their children. Beliefs about individual rights and obligations, family relationships, and the destiny of man are deeply rooted and cannot easily be shed, particularly if the alternatives do not seem viable or attractive. A Sikh grandfather, asked to give his consent to his grand-daughter's marriage to an English boy, who was liked and respected both by him and the rest of the family, expressed his agony of doubt and reluctance when he cried out: 'My beliefs are like my children. They are part of me. If I cast them aside or you take them away, I shall no longer exist.'

Since, when they feel criticized and threatened, immigrants are more likely to cling tenaciously to their own values and attempts to impose their own will—often quite inappropriately—social workers who hope to persuade immigrants to be more flexible need to be exceptionally careful to appreciate their point of view and their doubts and fears about change. The Khan case shows that this will often not be easy, since the very presence of a social worker can often seem a threat. Social workers must expect considerable hostility and antagonism from those who feel their ways of life are being seriously challenged.

Very occasionally, drastic steps, including court action, may be necessary to emphasize the seriousness of such behaviour as the continued severe chastizement of children. However, not surprisingly, immigrants, probably even more that natives, regard this as the ultimate proof of their failure to establish themselves successfully in a new country. They will need time to express their resentment of punishment which would be quite unlikely in their own countries, and a great deal of patient encouragement and support to survive such an experience.

Changes of custom and attitude inevitably mean pain and conflict which in our present society will be more acutely experienced by immigrants. Social workers must recognize that through the influence they bring to bear, they contribute to this. The greatest integrity is needed in deciding whether these demands are legitimate, as well as considerable courage, patience, and skill in coping with the inevitable anger and distress.

Cultural patterns or personal pathology?

There are occasions when social workers are at a loss to

know whether the behaviour or characteristics of the immigrants with whom they are working are manifestations of personal problems, towards which some help should be directed, or cultural patterns which are unfamiliar to the English. For example, does extreme passivity and resignation in the face of an imminent eviction or other crisis reflect a tradition of abandonment to Fate or Divine Providence, or is it a sign of acute depression? How far is the severe treatment of children or wives customary or a sign of a serious breakdown in relationships?

There are no easy ways of answering these questions, but social workers should not use their uncertainty as an excuse for absolving themselves of the responsibility to assess the problems that confront them as honestly and as carefully as they can. It can be helpful to try to discuss with the individuals concerned, or with their relatives and friends, the pattern of life in their native countries and the beliefs and philosophies on which it is built. Sometimes social workers need to be quite open about their confusion. If they decide to take the risk of intervening in situations about which they are uncertain, as sometimes they must, the reactions of the individuals concerned may give some clues as to the appropriateness of this course of action. Even when social workers are fairly sure that some behaviour reflects cultural traditions, as the previous section has indicated, there will be occasions when the consequences are serious enough to warrant intervention.

Working with immigrant families

Chapter 5 has shown that in their work with immigrants, social workers must bear in mind some unfamiliar conceptions of family life. With West Indians, the different family patterns, and the fairly fluid structure of some of these patterns means that care is needed in ascertaining who are the important members of a family network and what their respective roles are. The larger and often more rigid pattern of family life of Asian immigrants can also be confusing, in that social workers are uncertain about whom to approach and what pressures are brought to bear on individual members.

1 *Contact with relatives* When a family itself approaches a social work agency, or when it is referred by someone else, in the early stages of contact it is usually right for the social worker to consult the senior male members of an Asian family and to make sure that they have the opportunity of being included in any discussions about family problems. Social workers need not be too anxious that this wider network of consultation will be regarded as a breach of confidence in the same way as it would be in many English families. In extended and joint family systems, the affairs of individual members are usually common knowledge and a common concern.

There are, however, instances when social workers are approached by people for whom the traditional ways of managing and solving problems within a family are proving unsatisfactory. This may be especially true on the rare occasions that Indians and Pakistanis consult social work agencies. In these cases it could be extremely unwise to approach other members of the family before finding out exactly what the pressures are on the individual seeking help. Hutchinson (1969) has described some cases which include a Sikh girl's attempt to extricate herself from a marriage arranged by her family and a wife's efforts to leave her husband whom she regards as cruel and her unsuccessful attempt to establish herself independently from her family. In these circumstances the individuals concerned will clearly be most unwilling for their affairs to be discussed with other family members and may indeed express considerable fear of them. Lacking the personal resources to do this themselves, they may sometimes be trying to get social workers to extricate them from situations they now regard as intolerable, in the same way that parents often try to use social workers to exert the control over their children they feel they no longer possess themselves. Frequently, however, both these clients and the social workers may be pessimistic about their chances of settling happily outside the context of their family unless they can find an alternative protective environment.

These cases are extremely complex, and social workers may have to try to play for time while they form a more detailed picture of the life-style of the family concerned. How far it is still rooted in its native country? How many relatives are living in Britain? Do the members of the family intend to settle here or return home, and are they likely to carry out these intentions? How does the individual client fit into the family, and is he likely to find alternative satisfaction and protection outside it? Social workers may need to try to help their clients identify their alternative courses of action and their feelings about them, sometimes pointing out quite firmly that they will not be able to do more for an individual than he can do for himself. There will also be occasions when social workers will need to support the authority of a family over an individual who seems to need the protection and control of his relatives, while still holding open for him, and for the rest of the family, the possibility that he may eventually wish and need to be more independent. If a client does decide to break from his family, a social worker will be faced with considerable pressure from its members to restore him to his relatives. The social worker will also probably have to give the now isolated individual a great deal of practical and emotional support which will often only inadequately meet his needs.

In less serious cases it will usually be more appropriate to work within a family context, helping its members to bring into the open their distress about their strained relationships and their fears about the implications for the family as a whole. At times, the pressures of migration and the hardship of settling in Britain and the toll these take on family life may be bitterly resented. But many immigrants who feel they are only barely tolerated by the wider community are so socially insecure that they dare not express their negative feelings openly.

2 *Scapegoating* Bell and Vogel (1968) have observed that in these circumstances hostility and resentment may be kept within the confines of the family by being focused on one of its members, usually a child. In this way some solidarity and equilibrium are achieved and self-respect preserved. The behaviour of this scapegoat often reflects particular concerns of the family; social workers know of many cases where the misdemeanours of children and the wrath of their parents symbolize anxieties about achievement and recognition, and uncertainty about conflicting value systems. An example of this process is provided by the Khan family, whose youngest son, Hassan, might have become a scapegoat, had not his parents received some help with their anxieties. The process of scapegoating can sometimes be so vicious and destructive that a child may need some relief from his family if his self-confidence is to survive. However, since families often continue to try to solve their problems by projecting them onto one member, it is far more constructive if they can be helped to understand how they attempt to relieve their tensions and are given the security to do this in other ways.

3 *Marital relationships* Some social workers, particularly if they are young, find their work with immigrant families difficult, as they are influenced by their own conception of family life, with its relatively democratic structure and its emphasis on the importance and viability of individual self-assertion and independence. For those with no experience of life within a tight family network, it is easier to see the constraints this places on its members than its warmth and pleasures and the comfort and security of remaining in, or returning to, the fold, especially for

those immigrants who feel isolated in an alien and frequently unfriendly environment. Similarly, it is not easy for social workers, especially women, to appreciate the strengths and satisfactions of marital relationships in which the husband plays the more definite and dominant role, where love follows rather than precedes marriage, and where great importance and honour are attached to a wife's role as a mother and housewife. Too often, social workers involved with the marital difficulties of their immigrant clients, seeing a tangle of obedience and disobedience, submission, and sometimes physical control, fail to recognize that their perception of such a relationship is strongly influenced by fairly recent Western ideals of romantic love and the equality of husband and wife. They need, therefore, to take care to understand their immigrant clients' conception of marriage and of the possible solutions to their problems—and these may differ quite surprisingly from those of a social worker. In some areas immigrants themselves have established methods by which marital differences can be discussed and negotiated, and when the individuals concerned are in agreement, it can be helpful to use these.

4 The extended family and social work agencies

Now that we live in England we always have to remember that we are in a foreign country. If I alienate my wife or leave her, where shall I turn? Or if she is irritated with me, where can she go? ... We have no family here and if we start arguing and split up, what would become of our children? (Sharma, 1971, p. 65.)

There is a prevailing assumption amongst social workers, often well based, that immigrants are well able to cope with their problems within their own family network and that they would be quite indignant at the offer of social work help. There is, therefore, no need to make efforts to reach out to those immigrant families who do not come to social work agencies of their own accord. This view, if held strictly, ignores the fact that many families do not have kin in Britain, and that if they do, as chapter 4 has shown, the pressures of life in Britain frequently limit their capacity to support those outside their immediate family circle. Some families may, therefore, be greatly in need of help, while their ignorance of the social services, and possibly their embarrassment at their strange isolation, prevent their breaking into our welfare system. As in so many other cases, social workers should not always wait to be contacted, and in the absence of these approaches, assume there are no un-met needs. In the next decade, many immigrant families, who formerly would have relied on their own kin in crisis, will need the help of social work agencies. Social workers must be sensitive to the most appropriate ways of making their services known and of contacting families whose difficulties are compounded by the shame and shock of their isolation.

Probably more than in most families, a social worker will be seen by immigrants as an unwelcome intruder, with little idea of their way of life and the strains they are experiencing. He may also be seen as possessing fantastic degrees of power and influence. It can, therefore, be important for a social worker to adopt initially a fairly passive role, avoiding if possible too great an identification with any one family member which would alienate his relatives and might also blur his vision of its style of life. This can be an insecure and difficult role to play, but it is a necessary preliminary to being accepted as someone who has a contribution to make in the solution of family problems.

Working with immigrant organizations

Many social workers have been confused and disappointed by their contacts with immigrant organizations. They have expected a degree of consistency and an acceptance of responsibility for the welfare of immigrants with problems which is unrealistic given the divisions amongst immigrants and the emphasis they place on the responsibility of families to help their kin. Desai (1963) has described well the various aims of immigrant organizations and the pressures on them. The most successful are those which organize leisure facilities for immigrants, frequently on a commercial basis, such as Indian and Pakistani film associations, or the semi-political organization designed to protect and promote the interests of immigrant workers; even so, these groups are frequently subject to internal dissension which can reflect the political divisions of the immigrants' native countries. There may also be competition amongst different organizations drawing members from the same national group. Only recently have a few organizations emerged which are specifically concerned with the welfare of immigrants, and there are several which include the word 'welfare' in their name, but which would not see their role as helping individuals with personal or family problems.

It is, therefore, probably most useful for social workers to make their services known through some of the semi-commercial enterprises patronized by immigrants and to use their elaborate and extensive networks of communication. Through these organizations they may also be able to identify individuals who are able to help with specific immigrant problems. Sometimes such people emerge as semi-professional mediators who will negotiate for a family on a wide range of practical matters, including welfare problems. These 'middlemen' are often paid, either in money or in kind, by the families concerned. Social workers are sometimes uneasy about working with them, partly because of the financial arrangements, but also because they fear that even if they are meant only to be acting as interpreters, these 'middlemen' are not impartial, either in their presentation of their clients' problems and the social workers' comments and suggestions, or in the courses

of action they recommend. Although these are real difficulties, the use of paid middlemen needs to be seen as one
of the traditional and accepted ways by which families,
often illiterate and quite unfamiliar with the complexities
of urban life, conduct their affairs both in their native and
adopted countries. There may be few alternative ways for
social workers and immigrants to make contact with each
other, and since the 'middlemen' in immigrant communities
can be influential people, it can be more helpful for social
workers to make contact with them and to explain the
services they can offer, rather than to ignore or avoid them.

Some departments believe that they can bypass these
difficulties by employing immigrant social workers, and
clearly it is most useful to have on hand someone who
speaks some of the languages most commonly used by
immigrants. However, while it is most important for immigrants and coloured people to be represented in social work
agencies, as in all other areas of life, in most cases it
would not be appropriate for them to work only with
immigrant clients. Not only can such a policy be tinged
with ideas that only persons of a similar racial background
can understand and accept each other; it also underesti-
mates the extent to which immigrants can feel alienated
from and hostile to their more educated middle-class compatriots, perhaps believing that they will be treated by
them in the context of some of the more unsympathetic
traditions of their native countries.

Organizations concerned with the welfare of immigrants

In recent years a number of statutory and voluntary organizations have been formed whose aim is to promote the
interests of immigrants from the New Commonwealth and
their families. Details of some of these can be found at the
end of the final section of this volume. Some of these voluntary bodies cater mainly for immigrants of one national
group and may emphasize the importance of the mainten-

ance of cultural traditions and the need for the provision of self-help schemes, rather than reliance on the agencies of the Welfare State. Some of these ideals have developed against a background of growing mistrust of the impartial treatment of coloured people in Britain. At their most extreme, they stress the need for coloured people not only to accept their separation from the white majority, but to welcome and make use of this by forming cohesive groups which will support their members and take various measures to establish their rights. Apart from their important political role, such groups can have a valuable welfare function. Although some prefer to remain entirely separate from official organizations, others are willing to co-operate with them and welcome their support.

There is some confusion about the role of immigrant organizations. Their absence is frequently regretted, but when they emerge they are distrusted and discouraged if their aims and activities seem coloured by the expression of grievances and an emphasis on the necessity of protest and conflict if these are to be resolved. And yet it could be argued that such organizations truly reflect the circumstances and beliefs of at least some immigrants, who will be further alienated and drawn to more extreme positions if they are ignored by established agencies. The legislation and policies of official organizations have not been so liberal and consistent as to make it reasonable either to expect or insist on such ideals from voluntary organizations. The needs of many coloured people are so acute, and their future in Britain as problematic, that social workers cannot afford to ignore the possibilities of co-operating with any organization which could promote their welfare.

Prejudice and discrimination

Chapter 1 described briefly some of the origins of prejudice and the pressures which can lead people to discriminate against others. Lack of space prevents any extended discussion of the work social workers may need to undertake when faced with prejudice and discrimination, and only a few guide-lines can be mentioned.

It is relatively simple to reduce or remove the prejudice that arises from misunderstanding or ignorance. However, when this is associated with personality problems, it is unlikely to be influenced by rational argument or discussion. Equally, when prejudice is an expression of fears and insecurities which in themselves have a real basis, it is unhelpful to approach it directly. Attempting to arouse the guilt of prejudiced people by emphasizing their responsibility for weaker members of the community is nearly always unsuccessful. In a discussion of the dynamics of prejudice, Dicks (1959, pp. 37-38) writes:

> all these varieties of the prejudiced personality ... have in common an essential pessimism ... an expectation of deprivation rather than gratification ... at bottom these prejudiced persons cannot love life or their own and other people's goodness and worth ... it must be emphasised that these characters are not sick patients in the current sense but ordinary citizens.

Countless studies have revealed the actual or relative deprivation of millions of people who live in a highly stratified and competitive society; in this context, pessimism is a most natural response. In particular, in a vivid and most readable account of the despondency of the inhabitants of a Northern town, Seabrook (1971) has shown how easy it is for immigrants to become scapegoats for the woes of a community.

It is, therefore, usually more effective to approach the problem of prejudice indirectly, by focusing on, and taking seriously, those factors which contribute to the insecurity of individuals or groups. Sometimes only by relieving these is it possible to reduce tensions. By gaining the confidence of the more powerful but still insecure individuals, it is easier for them to identify the common problems they share with those towards whom they feel antagonistic, and to act in ways which will protect their own interests without destroying those of other people.

Social workers often find this more indirect approach extremely difficult, partly because they are alive to the hardships of minority groups which result from discrimination against them, but also because, in the controversies about the extent of prejudice and the need to control discrimination, they feel they should be above reproach, and are most sensitive about their own shortcomings in this area. Where indirect approaches are ineffective, and when immigrants are suffering because of prejudiced or discriminatory behaviour, social workers need to make their disapproval of this quite clear and, where appropriate, draw public attention to it and seek to control or modify its ill effects by other means. Nor should social workers forget that, to some extent, they have a role as leaders of humanitarian public opinion. There is good evidence that insecure people identify with strong leaders. There are many people who are prepared to feed and ignite their prejudices. Social workers have a part to play in combating this. In this context, as in so much of their contact with immigrants, social workers will find they have to tread an uncertain path. It may sometimes seem easier, but ultimately unethical and less effective, to avoid controversy in attempts to ingratiate themselves with everyone while succeeding in gaining the confidence of no one. They must not forget the moral nature of social problems. The words of Martin Luther King (1970, p. 10) are here deeply relevant:

It is again my deep conviction that ultimately a genuine leader is not a searcher for consensus, but a moulder of consensus. On some positions cowardice asks the question, 'Is it safe?' Expediency asks the question, 'Is it politic?' Vanity asks the question, 'Is it popular?' But conscience must ask the question, 'Is it right?' And there comes a time when one must take a stand that is neither safe, nor politic, nor popular. But one must take it because it is right.

Conclusion

The presence of immigrants throws into relief the values of the countries in which they have settled. Social work inevitably reflects these values and it can represent both the repressive rigidities of society as well as its more liberal and reforming elements. In their contact with immigrants, social workers will reveal their sensitivity and honesty in the understanding of problems, their imagination and resourcefulness in the help they give, their courage and skill in the handling of conflict, their generosity and compassion in the face of loneliness, confusion, and distress. Working with immigrants and their families brings social workers in touch with ambition, unselfishness, endurance, and courage. These are rare qualities. It is the privilege of social workers to be their witness.

Suggestions for further reading

Aspects of race relations

1 *Comparative studies and conceptual problems*

(a) Britain. Banton (1967), Richmond (1965), and Segal (1967) have published studies of race relations problems in several countries. Banton's book gives a good account of some of the major theoretical problems posed by the study of race relations and traces the history of attitudes towards racial differences. This is a major work and a useful text-book. Mason (1970) has written a good short introduction to the study of race relations. UNESCO (1969) have also published concise introductions to various aspects of the subject written by well-known authors. Rex's (1970) socio-logical analysis of race relations is most illuminating. Zubaida (1970) has edited a series of papers by major writers on race relations which provides a good introduc-tion to their longer works. In a stimulating article, Halsey (1970) discusses the future of race relations in the context of British reactions, in general, to social inequality.

The early settlement of coloured immigrants in Britain is described by Little (1947), Banton (1955, 1959) and Collins (1957). Garrard (1971) compares British reactions to Jewish and Commonwealth immigration. Foot (1971) discusses political attitudes to race and immigration in Britain. J. Brown (1970) gives an impressionistic but vivid account of the settlement in Bedford of several immigrant groups from Europe and the Commonwealth. He emphasizes the import-ance of cultural rather than colour differences in under-standing conflict both between different immigrant groups and between immigrants and natives.

(b) Israel. In a study of the settlement of immigrants in Israel, Eisenstadt (1954) provides a useful sociological framework for the analysis of immigration in modern societies.

(c) USA. The plight of the Negro in America and the racial problems facing American society are exhaustively discussed by Myrdal (1944). This long book is summarized and updated by A. Rose (1964). More recently, a report of the US Department of Labor (1965), commonly referred to as 'the Moynihan Report', discusses in detail the grave disruption in the Negro family, identifying this as one of the corner-stones in the dilemma of race relations in the USA. Goldschmid (1970) has edited some good research papers on the circumstances of black Americans. Several of these have a bearing on the situation of coloured people in Britain.

Carmichael and Hamilton (1969) have written a stimulating account of the background, aims, and ideals of Black Power. Martin Luther King's (1969) analysis of the Negro situation and the role of the Civil Rights Movement in the USA provides a powerful contrast.

2 *Prejudice and discrimination* The most concise accounts of the aetiology of prejudice and discrimination, published in pamphlet form, are by Hashmi (1967b) and Stafford-Clark (1967). Allport (1954) has written a classic study of the nature of prejudice, and Jahoda (1960) provides an interesting analysis of racial prejudice in largely psycho-analytic terms. This paper includes a discussion of the most effective ways of handling prejudice. Argyle (1970) summarizes briefly psychological interpretations of racial prejudice and Bloom (1971) writes about it in the context of social psychology. Rex and Moore (1967) underline the necessity of understanding discrimination in the context of the competition and conflict of urban society.

Statistics, legislation, and recent historical background

Major source books for information concerning all aspects of immigration and race relations in Britain have been published by E. J. B. Rose *et al.* (1969) and Patterson (1969). Rose's book is usefully updated and summarized by Deakin (1970). Field and Haikin (1971) have edited a comprehensive but concise collection of readings on aspects of immigration from the Commonwealth and the situation of coloured people in Britain. This book, which is most readable, is recommended as a simple short introduction to the study of race relations in the UK.

The statistics of immigration to Britain for the last hundred years are summarized by Cheetham (1972). The Institute of Race Relations publishes annually a useful booklet containing the most important and recent information concerning immigration from the Commonwealth. Eversley and Sukdeo (1969) have made a detailed study of the likely growth of the coloured population in Britain. Jones and Smith (1970) have studied the economic implications of Commonwealth immigration.

McDonald (1969) has written an account of English law as it affects race relations and immigration. It should be noted that there has been further legislation since this book was published. Lester and Bindeman (1972) provide a comprehensive guide to the Race Relations Acts and set these Acts in a historical and sociological context. Lester and Deakin (1967) edited a series of articles which discuss the policies necessary for the pursuit of racial equality.

Social circumstances of immigrants

1   *The urban environment and housing*   There is a considerable American literature documenting the sociology of inner city areas which became a magnet for the poor, including immigrants from rural areas, the Southern states, and Europe. A classic study was published by Park, Burgess,

and McKenzie (1925). This book was reissued in 1967. Emphasizing the distinction between peasant and urban society, Tönnies (1955), Redfield (1955), and Wirth (1964) underline the personal and family conflict experienced by most migrants to urban areas.

Rex and Moore's (1967) study of Birmingham draws attention most lucidly to the inherent conflict between different social groups arising from the demands of urban life, and the resulting pressures on the family, particularly the coloured migrant family. The analysis of the 'zone of transition' and the theory of 'housing classes' are vital to the understanding of the general development of race relations in Britain and the kinds of housing, employment, education, and welfare facilities available to immigrants. Rex has summarized this approach to the sociology of the inner city and its manifest and latent conflicts in a volume of readings edited by Pahl (1968).

Wilner, Walkley, and Cook's (1955) study of interracial housing projects in the USA throws an encouraging light on the development of relationships between white and coloured people housed in close proximity to each other.

2 *Education* Hawkes (1966), Burgin and Edson (1967), and Bowker (1968) have discussed some of the problems of the education of immigrant children. Power (1967) has written a concise account of various practices adopted by education authorities with large numbers of immigrant children. A report of the Department of Education and Science (1971) provides the most recent survey of the education of immigrant children and an account of appropriate policies and teaching methods. Kozol (1967) vividly describes the plight of children in American ghetto schools.

3 *Employment* Marsh (1967), Patterson (1968), Wright (1968), and McPherson and Gaitskell (1969) have discussed the employment most typically found by immigrants in Britain, the experiences of employers and employees, and

the problems connected with the employment of coloured people. Hepple (1970) writes excellently about racial discrimination in employment in Britain and the measures needed to counter this.

4 *Crime* Wolfgang (1966) has studied the incidence of crime amongst immigrants and different ethnic groups, and Bottoms (1967) has written an article which discusses the present crime rate amongst immigrants in Britain.

The social and cultural background of immigrants

The best and most readable account of the experiences of a family both before and after its migration is by Sharma (1971). This book consists of extracts from her lengthy conversations with an Indian family living in Britain. It provides a most vivid and moving description of the reactions and attitudes of many immigrants, whatever their ethnic background, and is probably the quickest and most enjoyable way of gaining insight into the predicament of the migrant family.

Oakley (1968) has edited a short book which includes concise accounts of the cultural background of the main coloured immigrant groups in Britain as well as a useful discussion of the problems they face. Morrish (1971) has written a more detailed and most helpful book on the same subject. Hall (1967) writes sensitively of some of the dilemmas facing coloured teen-agers in Britain. Evans (1971) surveys the attitudes of young immigrants.

1 *West Indians* The structure and circumstances of families in the West Indies have been studied by Blake (1953), R. T. Smith (1956), Kerr (1957), M. G. Smith (1965), Clarke (1966), and Henriques (1968). The most useful of these studies are those by Kerr and Clarke.

Fitzherbert (1967) has written a good summary of the main features of the West Indian family and their implications in migration. J. Smith (1971) describes the early history of West Indian boys coming to Britain after a period of separation from their parents. Calley (1965) discusses how the religious practices of West Indians in Britain reflect their philosophy and attitudes.

Glass (1960) and Patterson (1965) describe the early postwar settlement of West Indian immigrants in London. Glass includes a discussion of the various manifestations of racial friction in Britain, and Patterson provides a useful analysis of West Indian family life and social relationships in Britain. Most observers would agree that since these studies were made, the circumstances of West Indian immigrants have not improved, and, in some cases, have deteriorated; furthermore, the racial situation is now less fluid than it appeared to Glass and Patterson in the early 1960s.

2 *Pakistanis* There are few useful and accessible sources of information about Pakistanis in Britain. Hashmi (1967a) has written a short account of Pakistani family life, and Butterworth (1967a) has studied the life and social conditions of Moslem communities in England. A useful short account of the culture, politics, and history of Pakistan is provided by Stephens (1968). Guillaume (1964) describes the philosophy and institutions of Islam.

3 *Indians* Panikker (1960) has written a concise introduction to contemporary India. Ross (1961) provides an interesting and detailed description of the modern Hindu family in an urban environment. In two useful books, Desai (1963) and Aurora (1968) discuss the settlement in Britain of Gujarati Indians and Sikhs respectively. The Indian family in Britain is described briefly by Hiro (1967). Political and Economic Planning (1961) produced a paper which vividly describes the reactions of middle- and upper-class Indians to life in Britain. In a short book, Zinkin (1962) discusses the caste system.

The register of current research into various aspects of

race relations in Britain, published annually by the Institute of Race Relations, includes several studies which, when completed, will throw light on many of the questions raised in chapter 5 about the settlement of coloured immigrant groups in Britain.

4 *Other immigrant communities* Jackson (1963) describes the immigration of the Irish to Britain, and Gartner (1960) has studied the early Jewish settlement. Freedman (1955) has edited a series of papers on the contemporary Jewish community in Britain. Choo (1968) describes the Chinese community in London, and Tannahill (1958) has studied the post-war settlement of European workers in the UK. Zubrzycki (1956) gives an account of the Polish community in Britain.

Aspects of social work

1 *General issues* Moynihan (1969b), Sundquist (1969), and Townsend (1970) have edited useful books dealing with aspects of poverty and the measures taken to combat it. Morris and Rein (1967) and Moynihan (1969a) have described the contribution and limitations of community work programmes in the United States. These studies are most relevant to anyone interested in community action. The Calouste Gulbenkian report (1968) provides a good starting-point for the study of issues confronting British community workers. Halsey (1972) provides a clear analysis of the achievements and limitations of recent British educational priority programmes. In a useful series of short papers edited by Lapping (1970), well-known community workers discuss their current activities and preoccupations. Goetschius (1968) is one author who looks at ways of working for a consensus between different interest groups. This approach is criticized in an interesting article by Popplestone (1971).

Several studies, including those by Meyer *et al.* (1965),

Davies (1969), and Mayer and Timms (1970), have under-lined some of the limitations of casework. In a most lucid article, Perlman (1969) discusses the proper role and setting of this method of social work. Reid and Shyne (1969) have studied the respective merits of short- and long-term case-work. In a most original book, Caplan (1961) discusses preventive public health and social work programmes.

2 *Immigrants and social work* There is a dearth of literature which deals directly with those special problems of immigrant clients which are likely to be of immediate concern to social workers. Yudkin (1965), in a short pam-phlet, sensitively describes some of the needs of immigrant children, and Jackson (1971) reports on the growth of un-registered child minding and the West Indian community. Soddy (1961) has edited a book which includes some inter-esting contributions on the concepts of identity, values, and mental health in different cultural contexts.

Very little has been written which deals specifically with social work with immigrants. Leissner (1969) gives a vivid account of youth work in areas inhabited by a number of different, and frequently rival, ethnic groups. Kent (1965) has written an excellent article on aspects of the relation-ships between immigrants and social workers. Triseliotis (1963) has described some of the adjustment problems of immigrant school children; in a later article (1965), he dis-cusses the implications of cultural factors in casework with immigrants. He has also contributed a useful chapter to Oakley's (1968) book and has edited a useful collection of papers on aspects of social work with coloured immi-grants (1972). Raynor (1971) has studied the implica-tions of placing coloured children for adoption, and Kareh (1970) has written a short handbook designed especially for people interested in adopting a coloured child.

Amongst the wealth of literature on social work with families, very little refers specifically to immigrants. O. Pollak (1965b) has written an interesting article on the social determinants of family behaviour, and Parad and Caplan's (1965) framework for studying families in crisis can be usefully applied to the analysis of immigrant family problems. Some of the aims and techniques of conjoint family therapy are also relevant to work with immigrant families. Satir (1964) gives a good description of this method, and Skynner (1971) provides a brief introduction to it.

Personal accounts, autobiographies, and novels

Some of the most useful insights into the predicament of immigrants are to be gained from their autobiographies and accounts, real or imaginary, of their experiences in their new country. Selvon's novels (1956, 1965) provide a lively description of the life of newly arrived West Indian immigrants in London. Naipaul (1967) writes about the experiences of a middle-class migrant. Lamming (1953) gives a most sensitive account of a West Indian's attitude to his own culture and colour and his reaction to migration. He has also written about his own experiences as an immigrant (1960). Braithwaite (1959, 1962), another West Indian author, has described his experiences as a teacher and social worker in Britain.

Tajfel and Dawson (1965) have edited a series of essays which give a vivid account of the reactions of coloured Commonwealth students to Britain. In a collection of personal narratives and case studies Humphrey and John (1971) cast a sombre light on the experiences of coloured immigrants in Britain.

Baldwin (1970) and Cleaver (1970) are only two of the many Negro authors who have written powerfully of their experiences as black Americans in white society. Fanon (1970) provides a masterly philosophical and psychological analysis of the Negro's perception of the world.

Useful addresses

Statutory organizations

1 *The Community Relations Commission*

Russell Square House,
10/12 Russell Square,
London WC1B 5EH.

There are local community relations councils, partly sponsored by the C.R.C., throughout the country.

2 *The Race Relations Board*

5 Lower Belgrave Street,
London SW1W ONR.

The main work of the Board is undertaken by its regional conciliation committees.

3 *The U.K. Immigrants' Advisory Service*

St. George's Churchyard,
Bloomsbury Way,
London WC1A 25A

The U.K.I.A.S., which works in co-operation with voluntary agencies, deals with appeals against refusal of entry certificates to Britain and also gives welfare assistance to immigrants at the main ports of entry to the UK. The U.K.I.A.S. has regional offices in Birmingham, Bradford, Leeds, and Manchester.

216

Voluntary organizations

There are many voluntary organizations concerned with the welfare of immigrants. Some of the largest are:

1 *The Joint Council for the Welfare of Immigrants*

   Toynbee Hall,
   Commercial Street,
   London E1 6LS.

The J.C.W.I. assists Commonwealth immigrants and aliens —representing them where necessary—who are experiencing difficulties in connection with immigration control. It also gives welfare assistance to new arrivals in Britain.

2 *The Commonwealth Students' Children Society*

   Toynbee Hall,
   Commercial Street,
   London E1 6LS.

This society gives comprehensive assistance, including help with fostering arrangements and housing, to married overseas students and their families.

3 *The U.K. Overseas Students' Association*

   90 Buckingham Gate,
   London SW1W 0SS.

This organization offers assistance to students and will help with their problems over grants.

4 *West Indian Standing Conference*

   c/o Mr J. Hunte,
   Toynbee Hall,
   Commercial Street,
   London E1 6LS.

5 *National Federation of Pakistani Associations*

   41 Fournier Street,
   London E1 6QE.

Educational and research organizations

1 *The Institute of Race Relations*
   36 Jermyn Street,
   London SW1Y 6DT

The I.R.R. sponsors research studies into race relations and has published a large number of books dealing with this subject in a British context. The select bibliography (1967), register of current research studies, and Facts Papers are most useful.

2 *The Runnymede Trust*

   Stuart House,
   1 Tudor Street,
   London EC4Y OAD.

The Trust provides information about race relations in Britain. It publishes a monthly bulletin, sponsors research studies, and arranges courses.

Bibliography

ALLPORT, G. (1954). *The Nature of Prejudice*, Cambridge, Mass.: Addison-Wesley.

ARGYLE, M. (1970). *Psychology and Social Problems*, London: Methuen.

AURORA, G. S. (1968). *The New Frontiersmen: A Sociological Study of Indian Immigrants to the United Kingdom*, London: Hurst.

BAGLEY, C. (1968). 'Migration, Race and Mental Health', *Race*, vol. 9, no. 3.

—— (1969). 'A Study of Problems Reported by Indian and Pakistani Immigrants in Britain', *Race*, vol. 11, no. 1.

BALDWIN, J. (1970). *The Fire Next time*, London: Penguin.

BANTON, M. (1955). *The Coloured Quarter*, London: Cape.

—— (1959). *White and Coloured: The Behaviour of British People Towards Immigrants*, London: Cape.

—— (1967). *Race Relations*, London: Tavistock.

BARNARDO'S WORKING PARTY (1966). *Racial Integration and Barnardo's: Report*, Ilford: Barnardo's Homes.

BEETHAM, D. (1967). *Immigrant School Leavers and the Youth Employment Service in Birmingham*, London: Institute of Race Relations Special Series.

BELL, N. W. & VOGEL, E. G. (1968). *Modern Introduction to the Family*, London: Collier-Macmillan.

BENNINGTON, J. (1970). 'Community Development Project', *Social Work Today*, vol. 1, no. 5.

BILLINGSLEY, A. (1968). *Black Families in White America*, New York: Prentice-Hall.

BLAKE, J. (1953). *Family Structure in Jamaica*, Chicago: Free Press.

BLOOM, L. (1971). *The Social Psychology of Race Relations*, London: Allen & Unwin.

219

BIBLIOGRAPHY

BOTTOMS, A. E. (1967). 'Delinquency Among Immigrants', *Race*, vol. 8, no. 4.

BOWKER, G. (1968). *The Education of Coloured Immigrants*, London: Longmans.

BRAITHWAITE, E. R. (1959). *To Sir, With Love*, London: Four Square.

—— (1962). *Paid Servant*, London: Bodley Head.

BROWN, C. (1969). *Manchild in the Promised Land*, London: Penguin.

BROWN, J. (1970). *The Unmelting Pot*, London: Macmillan.

BURGIN, T. & EDSON, P. (1967). *Spring Grove: The Education of Immigrant Children*, London: Oxford University Press, for Institute of Race Relations.

BURNEY, E. (1967). *Housing on Trial*, London: Oxford University Press, for Institute of Race Relations.

BUTTERWORTH, E. (1967a). *The Muslim Community in Britain*, London: Church Information Office for the Church Assembly Board for Social Responsibility.

—— (ed.) (1967b). *Immigrants in West Yorkshire: Social Conditions and the Lives of Pakistanis, Indians and West Indians*, London Institute of Race Relations Special Series.

CALLEY, M. J. C. (1965). *God's People: West Indian Pentecostal Sects in England*, London: Oxford University Press, for Institute of Race Relations.

CALOUSTE GULBENKIAN FOUNDATION (1968). *Community Work and Social Change*, London: Longmans.

CAPLAN, G. (1961). *An Approach to Community Mental Health*, London: Tavistock.

CARMICHAEL, S. & HAMILTON, C. V. (1969). *Black Power*, London: Penguin.

CENTRAL ADVISORY COUNCIL FOR EDUCATION (1963). *Half Our Future* (Newsom Report), London: HMSO.

CÉSAIRE, A. (1955). *Discours sur le Colonialisme*, Paris: Présence Africaine.

CHEETHAM, J. (1972). 'Immigration', in Halsey, A. H. (ed.),

Trends in British Society since 1900, London: Macmillan.

CLARKE, E. (1966). *My Mother who Fathered Me*, London: Allen & Unwin.

CLEAVER, E. (1970). *Soul on Ice*, London: Panther.

COLLINS, S. (1957). *Coloured Minorities in Britain*, London: Butterworth.

COMMITTEE ON HOUSING IN GREATER LONDON (1965). *Report*, London: HMSO. Chairman: Sir Milner Holland.

COMMITTEE ON LOCAL AUTHORITY AND ALLIED PERSONAL SOCIAL SERVICES (1968). *Report* (Seebohm Report), London: HMSO (Cmnd. 3703).

CULLINGWORTH REPORT, see MINISTRY OF HOUSING AND LOCAL GOVERNMENT.

DAHYA, A. (1965). 'Pakistani Wives in Bradford', *Race*, vol. 6, no. 4.

DANIEL, W. W. (1968). *Racial Discrimination in England*, London: Penguin.

DAVIES, M. (1969). *Probationers in their Social Environment*, London: HMSO.

DEAKIN, N. (1970). *Colour, Citizenship and British Society*, London: Panther.

DEPARTMENT OF ECONOMIC AFFAIRS (1965). *The West Midlands—A Regional Study*, London: HMSO.

DEPARTMENT OF EDUCATION AND SCIENCE (1967). *Children and Their Primary Schools*, London: HMSO. Chairman: Lady Plowden.

—— (1971). *The Education of Immigrants*, London: HMSO, Survey of Education No. 13.

DESAI, R. (1963). *Indian Immigrants in Britain*, London: Oxford University Press, for Institute of Race Relations.

DEWEY, J. (1940). *Freedom and Culture*, London: Allen & Unwin.

DICKS, H. V. (1959). 'Psychological Factors in Prejudice', *Race*, vol. 1, no. 1.

EISENSTADT, S. N. (1954). *The Absorption of Immigrants*, London: Routledge & Kegan Paul.

BIBLIOGRAPHY

ELLIS, J. (1971). 'Fostering of West African Children', *Social Work Today*, vol. 2, no. 5.

ERIKSON, E. H. (1965). *Childhood and Society*, London: Penguin.

EVANS, P. (1971). *Attitudes of Young Immigrants*, London: Runnymede Trust.

EVERSLEY, D. & SUKDEO, F. (1969). *The Dependants of the Coloured Commonwealth Population of England and Wales*, London: Institute of Race Relations Special Series.

FANON, F. (1970). *Black Skin and White Masks*, London: Paladin.

FIELD, F. & HAIKIN, P. (eds.), (1971). *Black Britons*, London: Oxford University Press.

FITZHERBERT, K. (1967). *West Indian Children in London*, London: Bell.

FOOT, P. (1971). *Immigration and Race in British Politics*, London: Penguin.

FOREN, R. & BATTA, I. D. (1970). ' "Colour" as a Variable in the Use Made of a Local Authority Child Care Department', *Social Work*, vol. 27, no. 3.

FREEDMAN, M. (ed.) (1955). *A Minority in Britain*, London: Vallentine, Mitchell.

GARRARD, J. A. (1971). *The English and Immigration*, London: Oxford University Press, for Institute of Race Relations.

GARTNER, L. P. (1960). *The Jewish Immigrants in England 1870-1914*, London: Allen & Unwin.

GLASS, R. (1960). *Newcomers: The West Indians in London*, London: Allen & Unwin.

GOETSCHIUS, G. (1968). *Working with Community Groups*, London: Routledge & Kegan Paul.

GOLDSCHMID, M. L. (ed.) (1970). *Black Americans and White Racism: Theory and Research*, New York: Holt, Rinehart & Winston.

GOODMAN, M. E. (1964). *Race Awareness in Young Children*, London: Collier.

GUILLAUME, A. (1964). *Islam*, London: Penguin.

HALL, S. (1967). *The Young Englanders*, London: Community Relations Commission.

HALSEY, A. H. (1970). 'Thinking about Race Relations', *New Society*, 19 March.

—— (1972). 'Government Against Poverty in School and Community', in WEDDERBURN, D. (ed.), *Poverty, Inequality and Class Structure*, London: Cambridge University Press.

—— (1972). *Educational Priority*, London: HMSO.

HANDLIN, O. (1953). *The Uprooted*, London: Watts.

HASHMI, F. (1967a). *The Pakistani Family in Britain*, London: Community Relations Commission.

—— (1967b). *The Psychology of Racial Prejudice*, London: Community Relations Commission.

HAWKES, N. (1966). *Immigrant Children in British Schools*, London: Pall Mall Press, for Institute of Race Relations.

HENRIQUES, L. F. (1968). *Family and Colour in Jamaica*, London: MacGibbon & Kee.

HEPPLE, B. (1970). *Race, Jobs and the Law in Britain*, London: Penguin.

HILL, M. J. & ISSACHAROFF, R. M. (1971). *Community Action and Race Relations*, London: Oxford University Press, for Institute of Race Relations.

HIRO, D. (1967). *The Indian Family in Britain*, London: Community Relations Commission.

HOLMAN, R. (1968). 'Immigrants and Child Care Policy', *Case Conference*, vol. 15, no. 7.

—— (ed.) (1970). *Socially Deprived Families in Britain*, London: National Council of Social Service.

—— & RADFORD, E. (1969). 'Social Work in the Seventies', *British Hospital J. and Social Service Review*, 11 July.

HOOD, C. et al. (1970). *Children of West Indian Immigrants*, London: Institute of Race Relations Special Series.

HUMPHREY, D. & JOHN, G. (1971). *Because They're Black*, London: Penguin.

BIBLIOGRAPHY

HUNT REPORT, see YOUTH SERVICE DEVELOPMENT COUNCIL COMMITTEE.

HUTCHINSON, P. (1969). 'The Social Worker and Culture Conflict', *Case Conference*, vol. 15, no. 12.

INSTITUTE OF RACE RELATIONS (1970). *Facts Paper on the United Kingdom 1970-71*, London: Institute of Race Relations Special Series.

JACKSON, J. A. (1963). *The Irish in Britain*, London: Routledge & Kegan Paul.

JACKSON, S. (1971). *The Illegal Child Minders*, Cambridge: Priority Area Children.

JAHODA, M. (1960). *Race Relations and Mental Health*, Paris: UNESCO.

JENKINS, R. (1966). Address given by the Home Secretary to a meeting of Voluntary Liaison Committees, 23 May 1966, London: National Committee for Commonwealth Immigrants.

JOHN, A. (1970). *Race in the Inner City*, London: Runnymede Trust.

JONES, K. & SMITH, A. D. (1970). *The Economic Impact of Commonwealth Immigration*, London: Cambridge University Press.

KAREH, D. (1970). *Adoption and the Coloured Child*, London: Epworth Press.

KENT, B. (1965). 'The Social Worker's Cultural Pattern as it Affects Casework with Immigrants', *Social Work*, vol. 22, no. 4.

KERR, M. (1957). *Personality and Conflict in Jamaica*, London: Oxford University Press.

KING, M. L. (1969). *Chaos or Community?*, London: Penguin.
——— (1970). 'The Role of the Behavioral Scientist in the Civil Rights Movement', in Goldschmid, M. L. (ed.), op. cit.

KOZOL, J. (1967). *Death at an Early Age*, London: Penguin.

LAMBERT, J. R. (1970). *Crime, Police, and Race Relations*, London: Oxford University Press, for Institute of Race Relations.

LAMMING, G. (1953). *In the Castle of My Skin*, London: Michael Joseph.

—— (1960). *The Pleasures of Exile*, London: Michael Joseph.

LAPPING, A. (ed.) (1970). *Community Action*, London: Fabian Society.

LEISSNER, A. (1969). *Street Club Work in Tel Aviv and New York*, London: Longmans.

LESTER, A. & DEAKIN, N. (eds.) (1967). *Policies for Racial Equality*, London: Fabian Society.

LINDEMANN, E. (1965). 'Symptomatology and Management of Acute Grief', in PARAD, H. J. (ed.), *Crisis Intervention: Selected Readings*, New York: Family Service Association of America.

LESTER, A. & BINDEMAN, G. (1972). *Race and Law*, London: Penguin Books.

LITTLE, K. L. (1947). *Negroes in Britain*, London: Kegan Paul.

MCDONALD, M. (1969). *Race Relations and Immigration Law*, London: Butterworth.

MCPHERSON, K. & GAITSKELL, J. (1969). *Immigrants and Employment*, London: Institute of Race Relations Special Series.

MALCOLM X (1970). *Autobiography*, London: Penguin.

MARRIS, P. & REIN, M. (1967). *Dilemmas of Social Reform*, London: Routledge & Kegan Paul.

MARSH, P. (1967). *Anatomy of a Strike*, London: Institute of Race Relations Special Series.

MASON, P. (1970). *Race Relations*, Oxford: Clarendon Press.

MAYER, J. E. & TIMMS, N. (1970). *The Client Speaks*, London: Routledge & Kegan Paul.

MERTON, R. K. (1968). *Social Theory and Social Structure*, London: Collier-Macmillan.

MEYER, H. J., BORGATTA, E. F. & JONES, W. C. (1965). *Girls at Vocational High: An Experiment in Social Work Intervention*, New York: Russell Sage Foundation.

BIBLIOGRAPHY

MILNER HOLLAND REPORT, see COMMITTEE ON HOUSING IN GREATER LONDON.

MINISTRY OF HOUSING AND LOCAL GOVERNMENT (1969). *Council Housing: Purposes, Procedures, and Priorities*, London: HMSO.

MORRISH, I. (1971). *The Background of Immigrant Children*, London: Allen & Unwin.

MOYNIHAN, D. P. (1969a). *Maximum Feasible Misunderstanding*, London: Collier-Macmillan.

—— (ed.) (1969b). *On Understanding Poverty*, New York: Basic Books.

MYRDAL, G. (1944). *An American Dilemma*, New York: Harper.

NAIPAUL, V. S. (1967). *The Mimic Men*, London: André Deutsch.

NATIONAL ADVISORY COMMISSION ON CIVIL DISORDERS (1968). *Report*, New York: Bantam.

NEWSOM REPORT, see CENTRAL ADVISORY COUNCIL FOR EDUCATION.

NG KWEE CHOO (1968). *The Chinese in London*, London: Oxford University Press, for Institute of Race Relations.

OAKLEY, R. (1968). *New Backgrounds: The Immigrant Child at Home and School*, London: Oxford University Press, for Institute of Race Relations.

PAHL, R. E. (1968). *Readings in Urban Sociology*, London: Pergamon.

PANIKKER, K. M. (1960). *Commonsense about India*, London: Victor Gollancz.

PARAD, H. J. & CAPLAN, G. (1965). 'A Framework for Studying Families in Crisis', in PARAD, H. J. (ed.), *Crisis Intervention: Selected Readings*, New York: Family Service Association of America.

PARK, R. E., BURGESS, E. W. & MCKENZIE, R. D. (1967). *The City*, Chicago University Press.

PATTERSON, S. (1965). *Dark Strangers*, London: Penguin.

—— (1968). *Immigrants in Industry*, London: Oxford University Press, for Institute of Race Relations.

226

—— (1969). *Immigration and Race Relations in Britain 1960-1967*, London: Oxford University Press, for Institute of Race Relations.

PEACH, C. (1968). *West Indian Migration to Britain: A Social Geography*, London: Oxford University Press, for Institute of Race Relations.

PERLMAN, H. H. (1969). 'Can Casework Work?', in *Social Service Review*, vol. 42, University of Chicago Press, and in (1971) *Perspectives in Social Casework*, Pennsylvania: Temple University Press.

PLOWMAN, D. E. G. (1969). 'What are the Outcomes of Casework?', *Social Work*, vol. 26, no. 1.

PLOWDEN REPORT, see DEPARTMENT OF EDUCATION AND SCIENCE (1967).

POLITICAL AND ECONOMIC PLANNING (1961). *Indian University Students in Britain*. Issue of *Planning*, 13 November 1961, vol. 27, no. 456.

—— & RESEARCH SERVICES LTD (1967). *Racial Discrimination*, London: P.E.P.

POLLAK, M. (1970). 'A Comparative Study of the Development and Rearing of Three Groups of Three Year Olds', London: University M.D. Thesis (unpublished).

POLLAK, O. (1962). 'Cultural Dynamics in Casework', in C. KASIUS (ed.), *Social Casework in the Fifties*, New York: Family Service Association of America.

—— (1965a). 'A Family Diagnosis Model', in YOUNGHUSBAND, E. (ed.), *Social Work with Families*, London: Allen & Unwin.

—— (1965b). 'Social Determinants of Family Behaviour', in *ibid*.

POPPLESTONE, G. (1971). 'The Ideology of Professional Community Workers', *British Journal of Social Work*, vol. 1, no. 1.

POWER, J. (1967). *Immigrants in School: A Survey of Administrative Policies*, London: Councils and Education Press.

PRINCE, S. (1967). 'Mental Health Problems in Pre-School

West Indian Children', *Maternal and Child Care*, vol. 3, no. 26.

RAYNOR, L. (1971). *Adoption of Non-White Children*, London: Allen & Unwin.

REDFIELD, R. (1955). *The Little Community*, Chicago: Chicago University Press.

REID, W. J. & SHYNE, A. W. (1969). *Brief and Extended Casework*, New York: Columbia University Press.

REX, J. (1970). *Race Relations in Sociological Theory*, London: Weidenfeld & Nicholson.

— & MOORE, R. (1967). *Race, Community and Conflict*, London: Oxford University Press, for Institute of Race Relations.

RICHMOND, A. H. (1965). *The Colour Problem*, London: Penguin.

ROSE, A. (1964). *The Negro in America*, New York: Harper Torchbook.

ROSE, E. J. B. *et al.* (1969). *Colour and Citizenship: A Report on British Race Relations*, London: Oxford University Press, for Institute of Race Relations.

ROSS, A. D. (1961). *The Hindu Family in the Urban Setting*, Toronto: University of Toronto Press.

RUNNYMEDE TRUST (1970). *Race in the Inner City*, London: Runnymede Trust.

SATIR, V. (1964). *Conjoint Family Therapy*, California: Science & Behavior.

SEABROOK, J. (1971). *City Close-up*, London: Allen Lane.

SEEBOHM REPORT, see COMMITTEE ON LOCAL AUTHORITY AND ALLIED PERSONAL SOCIAL SERVICES.

SEGAL, R. (1967). *The Race War*, London: Penguin.

SELECT COMMITTEE ON RACE RELATIONS AND IMMIGRATION (1969). *The Problems of Coloured School Leavers*, London: HMSO.

—— (1970). *The Control of Commonwealth Immigration*, London: HMSO.

SELVON, S. (1956). *The Lonely Londoners*, London: Allan Wingate.

—— (1965). *The Housing Lark*, London: MacGibbon & Kee.

SHARMA, V. (1971). *Rampal and His Family*, London: Collins.

SINFIELD, A. (1969). *Which Way for Social Work?*, London: Fabian Society.

SIVANANDAN, A. (1967). *Coloured Immigrants in Britain: A Select Bibliography*, London: Institute of Race Relations Special Series.

—— & WATERS, H. (1970). *Register of Research on 'Commonwealth Immigrants' in Britain*, London: Institute of Race Relations Special Series.

SKYNNER, A. C. R. (1971). 'Indications for and against Conjoint Family Therapy', *Social Work Today*, vol. 2, no. 7.

SMITH, J. (1971). 'The Family History of West Indian Immigrant Boys', *British J. of Social Work*, vol. 1, no. 1.

SMITH, M. G. (1965). *The Plural Society in the British West Indies*, London: Routledge & Kegan Paul.

SMITH, R. T. (1956). *The Negro Family in British Guiana*, London: Routledge & Kegan Paul.

SODDY, K. (ed.) (1961). *Identity, Mental Health and Value Systems*, London: Tavistock.

STAFFORD-CLARK, D. (1967). *Prejudice in the Community*, London: Community Relations Commission.

STEPHENS, I. (1968). *The Pakistanis*, London: Oxford University Press.

SUNDQUIST, J. L. (ed.) (1969). *On Fighting Poverty*, New York: Basic Books.

TAJFEL, H. & DAWSON, J. L. (1965). *Disappointed Guests*, London: Oxford University Press, for Institute of Race Relations.

TANNAHILL, J. A. (1958). *European Volunteer Workers in Britain*, Manchester: Manchester University Press.

TÖNNIES, F. (1955). *Community and Association* (first published 1877), London: Routledge & Kegan Paul.

TOWNSEND, P. (ed.) (1970). *The Concept of Poverty*, London: Heinemann.

TRISELIOTIS, J. (1963). 'Immigrant School Children and their Problems of Adjustment', *Case Conference*, vol. 9, no. 7.

—— (1965). 'Casework with Immigrants: The Implications of Cultural Factors', *British Journal of Psychiatric Social Work*, vol. VIII, no. 1.

—— (1972). *Social Work with Colonial Immigrants and their Families*, London: Oxford University Press, for Institute of Race Relations.

UNESCO (1969). *Race and Science*, New York: Columbia University Press.

US DEPARTMENT OF LABOR (1965). *The Negro Family: The Case for National Action*, Washington, D.C.: Government Printing Office.

WILNER, D. M., WALKLEY, R. P. & COOK, S. W. (1955). *Human Relations and Interracial Housing*. Minneapolis: University of Minnesota Press.

WIRTH, L. (1964). *On Cities and Social Life*, Chicago: Chicago University Press.

WOLFGANG, M. E. (1966). 'Race and Crime', in KLARE, H. (ed.), *Changing Concepts of Crime and its Treatment*, London: Pergamon.

WRIGHT, P. (1968). *The Coloured Worker in British Industry*, London: Oxford University Press, for Institute of Race Relations.

YOUTH SERVICE DEVELOPMENT COUNCIL COMMITTEE (1967). *Immigrants and the Youth Service*, London: HMSO. Chairman: Lord Hunt.

YUDKIN, S. (1965). *The Health and Welfare of the Immigrant Child*, London: Community Relations Commission.

ZINKIN, T. (1962). *Caste Today*, London: Oxford University Press, for Institute of Race Relations.

ZUBAIDA, S. (1970). *Race and Racialism*, London: Tavistock.

ZUBRZYCKI, J. (1956). *Polish Immigrants in Britain: A Study of Adjustment*, The Hague: Nijhoff.

Printed in the United States
by Baker & Taylor Publisher Services

Printed in the United States
by Baker & Taylor Publisher Services